JASON: 1

STIGMA: 0

JASON: 1
STIGMA: 0

My battle with mental illness at home and in the workplace

Dear Peter,

JASON W. FINUCAN

Jason

Bell Let's Talk

2020

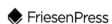

FriesenPress

Suite 300 - 990 Fort St
Victoria, BC, V8V 3K2
Canada

www.friesenpress.com

Copyright © 2019 by Jason W. Finucan
First Edition — 2019

Cover Photo: Fany Ducharme, www.fanyducharme.ca

ISBN
978-1-5255-4462-0 (Hardcover)
978-1-5255-4463-7 (Paperback)
978-1-5255-4464-4 (eBook)

1. SELF-HELP, DEPRESSION

Distributed to the trade by The Ingram Book Company

TABLE OF CONTENTS

DISCLAIMER

This book contains details of my personal experience with mental illness, specifically, bipolar disorder and the stigma surrounding it. It is the story of one person and is in no way intended to represent the experience of every person who faces mental illness and stigma. Individuals experience mental illness in their own unique way, to varying degrees of severity and with varying degrees of success with respect to treatment. In addition, the details shared regarding my medical treatment are in no way medically prescriptive for any other person. Readers experiencing mental illness should always consult their physician prior to taking any medication.

My intention in writing this book is to help open people's minds to the realities of mental illness and stigma in our society today, and ideally provide some measure of hope for those currently facing this challenge. I have expertise on this topic as a result of personal experience with mental illness, management experience, extensive academic research, and years of delivering training and keynote lectures on this topic. Mine is only one perspective, however, and there is a vast array of resources available at the international, national, and local levels (see the recommended resources section at the end of this book for a full list). I encourage you to research as much as you can so you fully understand how mental illness may be affecting your life, or that of your loved one or colleague.

Finally, if you are reading this and experiencing suicidal thoughts, please know these two truths: **you have value, and there is help available**. Please search for crisis, help, or suicide hotlines in your area.

DEDICATION

For Anna, who didn't flinch when, on our second date, I shared that I had bipolar disorder. Amazingly free of stigma, you stayed and became the best friend, partner, caregiver, and wife a man could possibly hope for.

This book, my company StigmaZero, and so many of the things I cherish in my life would have never happened were it not for you, my Polish Princess.

Thank you, and I love you. You are my favorite.

PROLOGUE

Mental illness is unfair. It can tear apart relationships, ruin careers, and, in the most tragic instances, end lives. But there's one aspect of mental illness that makes it even worse for everyone whose lives it touches: *stigma*.

According to the Oxford Dictionary, stigma is defined as "a mark of disgrace associated with a particular circumstance, quality, or person." It gives the synonyms "shame, disgrace, dishonour, humiliation, and bad reputation."

In this context, stigma is the unwanted complication accompanying mental illness that doesn't come with other major illnesses, such as cancer or heart disease. Although stigma makes mental illness especially unfair and devastating, it is something we have the power to change.

I learned this the hard way—through direct personal experience— over many years. I faced a major heart defect at nine years old, and later, bipolar disorder. By comparing the two experiences, both personally and professionally, I realized the destructive power of stigma.

I wrote this book, in which I share many of my stories and lessons learned, with one goal in mind: that you may learn from my mistakes and successes, as well as my misfortune and luck, to help eradicate stigma from our lives and workplaces. A key conclusion I have come to is this: the stigma is, in fact, worse than the illness itself.

It is devastating to experience the symptoms of a mental illness, and even more so to be officially diagnosed with one. In that way, there is no difference when compared with a physical illness such as cancer. However, unlike cancer, a diagnosis of mental illness is quickly followed by internal and external stigma, which profoundly worsens the situation.

Despite significant gains in this area in recent years, stigma still surrounds mental illness, causing a lingering lack of empathy and understanding. All too often, blatant discrimination results. This stigma, and all that comes with it, is inappropriate, unnecessary, and offensive. It causes so much additional pain, and, even worse, it creates delays in people seeking help when they experience a mental illness. This, in turn, leads to significant delays in diagnoses and treatment strategies. Most tragically, this increases the number of people who die by suicide each year.

We have the power to change all of this by ending the stigma. Read on to find out how, and let's get rid of it together.

Jason Finucan
January 2019

HOW TO USE THIS BOOK

I have organized this book so you can read it from start to finish, if you wish. You can also read it in segments according to your need or interest. If you have picked it up because you want to learn more about a particular mental illness, such as depression, you might start with the chapter on depression. If you want to understand stigma and how to tackle it in your own life, the chapters on stigma are for you.

If you are an executive, HR professional, or manager, and you want to learn strategies to tackle stigma in the workplace, then pay special attention to the six "Create Your StigmaZero Workplace" segments found throughout this book.

Regardless of why you are reading it, I hope that, in some small way, the messages in this book make you feel empowered to join the growing movement to end the stigma of mental illness.

CHAPTER 1
PHYSICAL ILLNESS

TWO HUNDRED BEATS PER MINUTE

Each day after my grade four class let out, my brother and I would head home and watch our favorite TV show, *Three's Company*. I'd grab a bowl of cereal, sit cross-legged on the floor in front of the TV, and laugh as I watched the antics of Dave, Janet, Chrissy, and Larry. In general, I was a happy nine-year-old boy, and this ritual was one of my favorite parts of the day.

One day, however, everything changed.

As I sat on the floor, my heart abruptly started to beat so fast, it seemed like it might burst. Terrified, I called out to my dad: "DAD! SOMETHING'S WRONG WITH MY HEART!" He rushed over to me, confused and helpless, and when he felt how fast my heart was racing, his face went white. His reaction showed me how scary the situation was. Dad was always extremely calm under pressure; in fact, the more serious a situation, the calmer his response. This time, I couldn't help but notice his look of panic.

This frightening moment is seared into my memory. My heart, which I'd never paid any attention to, was beating so fast, it was actually causing me pain. My dad scooped me up, told my brother to get ready, and rushed me to the hospital. However, on the way there, my heart rate suddenly returned to normal. The doctors were not able to diagnose the problem without it occurring as they tested me.

This became a strange routine. Whenever my heart raced, we hopped in the car and headed to the hospital, but then my heartbeat would return to normal along the way. After several frustrating visits, all of which resulted in perplexed doctors unable to put their finger on the problem, we stopped going to the hospital altogether. We would just go for a drive, as it seemed the car ride itself stopped the attack.

During these attacks, I would be conscious but in terrible discomfort. My heart would race two hundred beats per minute, and my blood pressure would spike severely. The combination made me feel dizzy and faint, with extreme pressure in my chest and neck. I was unable to stand; my only option was to lie down and wait it out.

One of the most confusing aspects was that the attacks would start out of nowhere and for no apparent reason. Sometimes they happened when I was playing road hockey, and sometimes when I was at rest. Sometimes they occurred during the day when I was at school, and sometimes late in the evening. They lasted between twenty and forty-five minutes, which feels like an eternity when one's heart is pounding that hard.

From the time of that first attack while watching *Three's Company*, I experienced an average of two attacks a week; the next one was always a constant threat in the back of my mind.

After nearly a year of living in this terrible limbo, I finally caught a break that led to a diagnosis.

My parents had divorced a few years earlier, and I was living with my dad and one of my two brothers near Orillia, Ontario. Orillia is a city of 35,000 people, located on the shores of two small lakes an hour and half north of Toronto. My mom had relocated to Toronto, and she suggested we change my family doctor to one in the city. This proved to be a smart move.

Upon hearing of my track record of symptoms, my new GP ran an electrocardiogram (ECG) test on me. Looking at the results, he immediately referred me to a heart specialist at Toronto Hospital for Sick Children, also known as SickKids Hospital. That led to more tests and a consultation with a heart specialist, who advised my mom and me what was wrong with my heart. After all this time, we finally had a diagnosis: I had a rare nerve defect in my heart called Wolff-Parkinson-White (WPW) syndrome.

This doctor explained that WPW syndrome is an extremely rare defect in the nerves that initiate each heartbeat. This defect allows for, in a sense, a "short circuit" in the electrical current running through those nerves. It resulted in acute tachycardia, which in my case meant a suddenly and violently elevated heart rate. He said that not only was WPW rare, but the form I had was the rarest form. It was, in fact, unusual for a human heart to reach the speed that mine did. It was also unusual for the attacks to cause the pain and discomfort I experienced.

I felt like I had won a sort of "reverse lottery," but my self-pity was short lived. After years of confusion, I was just happy we finally had clarity about what was wrong with my heart. And more importantly, we had options for treatment.

We learned there was a chance WPW syndrome could be treated with medication, but the only way to fully correct it was with open-heart surgery. We tried the medication, which was supposed to reduce the occurrences and severity of the attacks. But by the time I was in grade seven, it became clear the treatment wasn't working. I was continuing to have at least two attacks a week, which were dramatically affecting my life at school, as well as my personal life. I was forced to lie down as soon as possible after an attack began. That meant having to leave class or suddenly stop playing games during recess.

I realized I didn't want to continue living like that if a solution was available, and my frustration grew. Even at twelve years old, I began to view open-heart surgery as the lesser of two evils, so I asked my mom, dad, and the heart specialist at SickKids if we could schedule the surgery. I still remember the look of surprise on my doctor's face as he realized this request was coming from me, not my parents. He actually dropped his pen and stared at me for a long moment, totally shocked. He said he had never seen a young patient request an optional surgery in this way.

As it turned out, the years of dealing with this heart defect had made me a very old young man.

MY OPEN-HEART SURGERY

As you might imagine, it took time to schedule a major heart surgery. We made the request in October 1987, and within a few weeks, we were given a date: April 12, 1988. While I felt relieved knowing the surgery was booked, it was still a challenge for me to wait nearly six months.

At first, I could put things out of my mind fairly easily and just live my life. However, as "D-Day" (as I called it) approached, I became more and more scared. Although still young, I fully understood how serious this surgery would be. The four to six weeks leading up to the surgery were incredibly difficult and anxiety-filled.

D-Day finally came. While the operation was scary, I was fortunate to come out of it with a repaired heart and, after a long recovery, my full health. There was a fifty percent chance I'd need a pacemaker, depending on how the procedure went. However, my surgeon and the surgery's success spared me that fate. I am eternally grateful for the extraordinary staff members in the heart ward of SickKids for their exceptional work with me.

Throughout the process were many memorable experiences I still remember with clarity after all these years—and will never forget.

Steve—Like a Friend and Brother to Me

Steve (not his real name) was my hospital roommate. He was four years older than me, sixteen at the time, and he was very, very sick. Unlike my nerve defect that wasn't life threatening and could be surgically repaired, Steve had a complex vascular problem in his heart. He was scheduled for surgery shortly after mine, but I learned it wasn't going to cure him.

When it became clear to me that Steve was extremely ill, I asked my nurse about him while he was out of the room for tests.

"Is Steve going to be okay?"

My nurse looked at me with kind, sad eyes and told me the truth. "No, dear. He is very sick. He likely won't be leaving this hospital."

As I got to know Steve, I was amazed by his positive attitude. He was funny, loved to joke around, and never seemed to despair about his health. I don't know if he knew he may have only a short time to live, but if he did, he never let it show. He took great interest in me and my situation, and since he had experienced surgeries before, he offered advice on what I should expect. His generosity and kindness were nothing short of amazing, especially given his tragic situation. In just a few days, I felt like I had a new friend and even another older brother.

I shared that room with Steve for the days leading up to my surgery, but when I returned from post-op and intensive care, he was gone. I never found out exactly what happened, but based on the nurses' comments, it seemed that Steve had succumbed to his illness. Although I was facing my own recovery, I was sad to think my friend had died. How unfair that my illness could be fixed while his couldn't.

It's easy to feel sorry for yourself when you're sick at any age, but especially when you are twelve. You wish you could just be normal like all your classmates. You wish you didn't have to go through all this. But I managed to avoid wallowing in self-pity, mostly because of the way my parents had raised me. And because of Steve.

In fact, meeting Steve became one of the experiences from my time at SickKids that dramatically affected me for the rest of my life. Instead of self-pity, I was filled with empathy, sadness, and gratitude. I felt empathy for Steve's misfortune in having such a serious illness. I felt sad that he was taken so young. At the same time, I felt enormous gratitude that I was alive, that my heart was repaired, and that I didn't need a pacemaker.

I deliberately thought I would always appreciate my health and my life, and I would never forget Steve and all the other sick kids who didn't have the privilege of leaving the hospital and recovering their health. That sense of gratitude has never left me—and would later save my life.

Mapping the Nerves to My Heart Pre-op

The procedure to map the nerves in my heart in preparation for surgery was a memorable experience. They called it a "catheterization," because it required a catheter to be inserted into a main artery in my groin. This catheter was fed to my heart, and a slight electrical current was used to trigger an episode of tachycardia. What made this so memorable—and frankly awful—was that I had to be awake for the entire ninety-minute procedure. Before this, I had never experienced an episode lasting more than forty-five minutes. This proved to be the longest ninety minutes of my young life.

I had to lie on a table with my arms and legs tied down, which was necessary to keep me still and allow for precise mapping. The attacks were extremely uncomfortable, and as they progressed past thirty minutes, they became downright painful. I could feel the veins in my neck throbbing from the pressure, I felt dizzy and, eventually, nauseated. I had to endure an attack of twice the duration I had ever experienced before. Up to that point in my life, I can easily say it was the biggest challenge I had ever faced.

Two days later, it would be eclipsed by a new challenge.

Floating into the Operating Room

An hour before my surgery, a nurse offered me a small pill that she said would calm my nerves. I didn't ask what it was, and to this day, I still have no idea. I took the pill, grateful for anything to lessen the abject fear I was feeling.

Not long after taking it, I felt the effects of the drug—and they were spectacular. Not only did I feel zero fear, but I was actually quite giddy. It seemed as though I was floating on my bed, and my vision produced long, smoky trails behind anything that moved. While my bed was being rolled down the hallway to the operating room, I felt like I was on a ride, all the time being mesmerized by the lights on the ceiling drifting by.

Once outside of the operating room, I was told we'd need to wait a few minutes before going in. I honestly didn't care, because now when people walked by, I was seeing trails *and* hearing a cool "vrroomm" sound. Thoroughly entertained, I didn't have a care in the world.

A few minutes later, though, I experienced the equivalent of a cold shower to snap me out of it. As I was rolled into the operating room (OR) and moved onto the main operating table, the reality of the situation brought me crashing down to earth. Here's what I noticed right away.

First, it was freezing. The OR is kept very cool, and I was nearly naked. I instantly started shivering.

Second, I was given a minute to look around. I wish I hadn't been. I noticed an array of shiny, sharp tools laid out on a tray. They included scalpels, clamps, and more tools that I couldn't identify. And then I looked up and saw something both amazing and frightening. Hanging from the ceiling above the operating table was a circular saw. It looked like the kind of saw I had seen in wood shop, although much cleaner and with a finer blade.

I realized the saw was to cut my breast bone to access my heart. I must have looked a little green because the anesthesiologist approached me right then and said in a calm voice, "I think it's time for you to go to sleep now."

"Okay," I replied. "Should I count backwards from ten?"

He smiled and said, "If you like." So I tried. I think I managed to say "ten, nine …" and that was it. Blackness.

Surreal Post-op Complications

Thankfully, I don't remember a thing from the surgery itself, although I do recall waking up in intensive care. It was a surreal experience for several reasons.

First, being on a ventilator is incredibly disorienting, because I wanted to breathe on my own, but I was too weak. Every few seconds, my lungs filled with air automatically. The sensation of all the tubes and wires intruding into my body only added to the discomfort.

Second, the pain medication (in my case, morphine) was extremely strong and left me feeling dazed and disoriented.

Finally, I had a very high fever and could tell that bags of ice were placed around my head. Overall, I felt awful, but thankfully I was only conscious for short bursts of time.

Having a fever as well as difficulty coming off the morphine and breathing on my own proved challenging. These complications extended my stay in intensive care to four days instead of the planned twenty-four to thirty-six hours. I was unconscious for most of that time; it would have been unbearable had I been awake for more than a few hours of that time.

One of my few clear memories in intensive care came thanks to a visit from my oldest brother. He had always hated hospitals, so it was a pleasant surprise to wake up and see him standing over me. However, he looked awful—stressed, worried, and uncomfortable being there. I felt sorry for him.

If I had been able to speak, I would have thanked him for coming and told him it was okay if he needed to leave. However, one of the side effects of being on a ventilator is that you can't speak at all. He leaned in and looked closely at me, then turned to my mom and asked, "Why are his eyes so glossy?" I thought that was funny, and then I was out again.

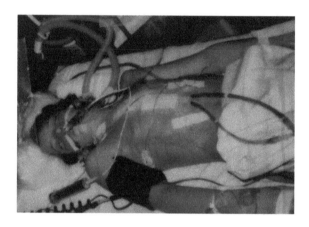

This photo was taken on April 13, 1988, the first of my four days in intensive care. I had a high fever, which is why bags of ice can be seen around my head. The dark stains on my body look like blood, but they're actually iodine from the operation.

On the Road to Recovery

After my time in intensive care, I had one more major challenge to overcome. I was finally off the ventilator and morphine, and my fever had broken, but I was in extreme pain and breathing with difficulty. I was placed in a holding room for one day and had access to oxygen; however, the doctors said I couldn't use it all the time. I had to learn how to breathe on my own again. I was also put on a schedule of pain medication, and my next shot of Demerol never seemed to come soon enough.

In extreme pain and gasping for each breath with only short bursts of relief, those twenty-four hours seemed like an eternity. In a situation like that, to quote one of my favorite movies, *The Shawshank Redemption*, "…time draws out like a blade."

Finally, I began breathing normally, and the pain slowly subsided. I was moved back to my original room to continue my recovery until my discharge just over a week later. The time passed without further complications, and I could feel my body improving with each passing day.

The following photos show how happy and grateful I was. After all, I was alive; I had a healthy heart and no pacemaker; I was on the path to recovery and a life without tachycardia; and I was showered with love, empathy, and support from my family and my friends from school. In fact, every single one of my classmates wrote me a get-well letter, and friends from my previous school sent me a hand-drawn card. I treasure them to this day.

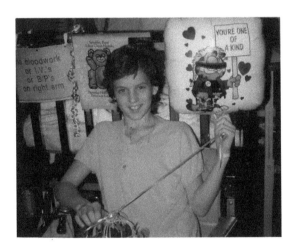

This photo is a powerful reminder of the impact of empathy—and zero stigma—on a person facing a major illness. I am genuinely happy here, despite having just gone through the worst experience of my life up until then.

The following three images are of the hand-drawn card I received from the students of my previous school. I am so touched they took the time to send this to me; I hadn't been a student at that school for nearly three years! The support rallying around me was incredible.

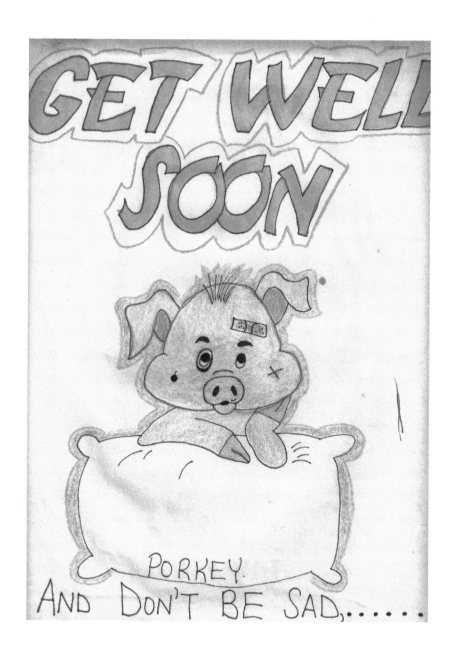

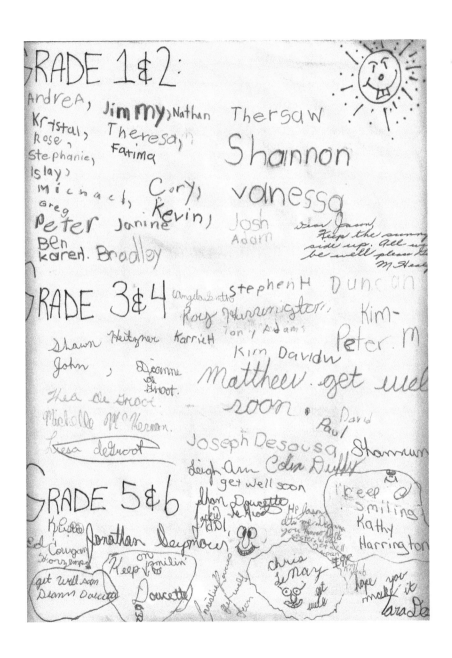

GRADE 1&2:

Andrea, Jimmy, Nathan   Thersaw
Kristal, Theresa,
Rose,   Fatima   Shannon
Stephanie,
Islay,   vanessa
Michael, Cory,
Greg   Kevin,   Josh
Peter Janine   Adam
Ben
Karen. Bradley

Dear Jason,
Keep the sunny
side up. All will
be well please ...
M. Healy

GRADE 3&4   Angela Smith Stephen H Duncan
             Roy Harrington,   Kim-
Shawn Heitzner KarrieH Tony Adams Peter. M
John ,   Deonne   Kim David
          de Groot. Matthew. get wel
Thea de Groot.   soon.
Michelle McKernan.   Paul David
Lesa deGroot   Joseph Desousa Shannum
                Leigh Ann Colin Duffy
GRADE 5&6   get well soon
                John Doucette   Keep
Kristie   Jackie Le Nod He Jason smiling
Ed Corrigan Jonathan Seymour   Kathy
  Korzemp   Harrington
get well soon Keep on smilin' chris
Dianna Doucette Doucette   Le May hope you
                                       make it
                                       Tara De...

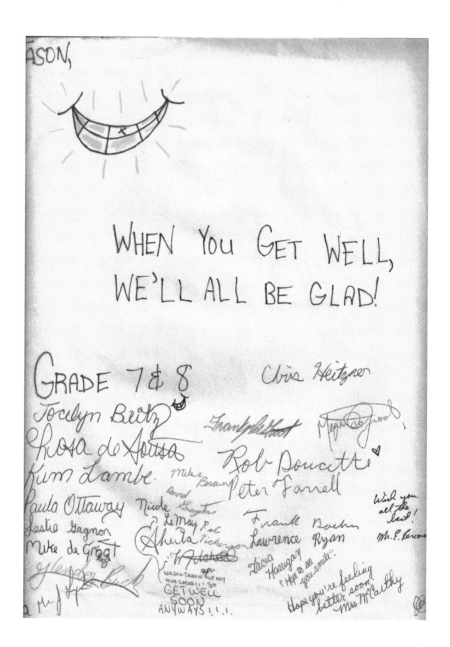

The following images are two of the more than thirty letters I received from my grade seven classmates while I was in the hospital recovering from surgery. Our teacher, Mr. O., had informed the class of my heart problem and surgery only after I left class on the day I was admitted to the hospital. Until that point, my heart condition had been kept a secret; my classmates knew I had some sort of health condition, but they didn't know what it was, or that it would require surgery. After informing the class, Mr. O. gave the students the opportunity to write me a letter, and to my surprise, they all did. Their letters were thoughtful, kind, supportive, and funny. It meant the world to me to receive such support.

These two letters are from my two closest friends from that time, Clara and Marc. I am still in contact with them, and they gave me permission to share them here.

Dear Jason   april 20/88

        Hi how are you? I'm alright.
God I hate writing letters, almost
as much as I hate mixing batter
in homeec. Speaking of homeec.
we made choccolate chip cookies
(as they were called.) They were
all right, just a tad different.
Mo O enjoyed them! (he ate 8 of
them!) Now he gained weight so
he said "If anyone catches me
eating anything in class I'll pay
you 20$ on the spot!" those words
exactly. So keep an eye on him
when he comes to see you!

We've been dancing our little hearts
out lately. (now waltzing) Well
nothing exciting is happening in
class except, for me passing the
math test (with an A+) So maybe
I do still have a chance of being
a nerd (like some people I know!)
I even passed the science, and boy
was my mom was shocked!

Everyone hopes you get better really
soon. We all miss you a lot! The
class isn't the same with out you
(and your tight jeans!) Well I
better stop writing before I bore
you to sleep! I'll be seeing you
real soon. So you better get better
(cause you'll be better off!) I love
the word better!
                        love your really
                        good friend Elana!

P.S. go ahead, pick
        out all the spelling mistakes!

22 Grovenest Dr.
Ont. M1F-4J3
April 18/88

Dear Jason

Hi, how have you been?, alright I hope.
anyhow, I was really surprised when Mr "O"
explained where you were going and what
was wrong. I always knew you had to
take sleeping pills, and sometimes I saw you
get up and walk out of the classroom
without permission, but I never thought
anything of it. Now I find out it was
something as serious as this.
   I was going to tell you about Mr "O"
"surprise party" and how unselfish it
was, but I figuer everbody else is writing
about it so I will start on something more
personnal. I heard you asked out Clara
well I hope she says yes to you, well
finally I want to say that the classroom has not been the same lately
and I have kind of been sad and
thinking alot about you and I have
come to a conclusion. You are a great
friend and I really think you are
neat.   hope to see you soon
                             from Marc Reynolds

ZERO STIGMA DEFINED

I still feel overwhelmed by the love, empathy and support I received during those difficult years, which were defined by my heart defect and subsequent surgery.

Not once did anyone treat me like I had done something wrong.

Not once did my family or friends seem uncomfortable with my illness.

Not once did my teachers question my motivation or work ethic when they learned I had to miss more than two months of school as I recovered from surgery.

I was allowed to face this challenge with absolutely zero stigma from those around me. I had no idea how lucky I was that stigma wasn't a part of my experience.

At the time, it all seemed normal. And it was. I had every reason to expect I'd be supported and loved and rallied around during this time. Why would anyone doubt, judge, or discriminate against me for a heart defect and the limitations it placed on my life? Why would anyone blame me or question my strength of character or work ethic? That would have been unacceptable to everyone, perhaps even ridiculous.

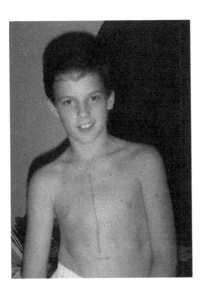

This photo was taken at my home in Toronto, Ontario, Canada, shortly after being released from SickKids Hospital in late April 1988.

As this photo shows, I wasn't made to feel embarrassed by my new (and rather huge) scar. My family photographed me this way in part to remind me that the scar didn't take anything away from who I was. I was still me; in fact, I had become special.

We even made jokes about how I could make up stories about the scar, like a knife fight while heroically saving someone. My facial expression doesn't show any effects of stigma or judgment; instead, it exudes a sense of pride.

Without any of us realizing it, something else was happening as well. The complete absence of stigma during my experience with this major physical illness unwittingly set the stage for a deep understanding of what stigma is and why it occurs. This would prove life-changing years later, when I suddenly experienced the symptoms of a mental illness.

The two experiences couldn't have been more different.

CHAPTER 2
MENTAL ILLNESS

CREATE YOUR
STIGMAZERO WORKPLACE
PART 1

Staggering Statistics:
How One in Four is Really Four in Four

You've likely heard this statistic: *One in four people will experience a mental illness in their lifetime.* The sources include the World Health Organization (WHO), the Canadian Mental Health Association (CMHA), the National Alliance on Mental Illness (NAMI), and others. And although it sounds frightening, this statistic has proven to be true for years.

Given the negative effect mental illness can have on a person's career and personal life, one in four, or twenty-five percent, is a staggering percentage. But I must be the bearer of bad news. The real statistic is four in four. *Everyone* is affected. It's not only the person who falls ill with symptoms; everyone in the person's immediate social and professional circles is affected.

How are people affected by mental illness even when it doesn't occur in them? Let's consider this example. When a colleague, manager, or direct report begins showing symptoms of a mental illness, such as depression, it can be confusing to know why the person's behavior has changed. He or she could have self-stigma and be in denial about the illness. This might cause the person to fall into the trap of *presenteeism*—that is, attempting to work while dealing with an illness, often at significantly reduced capacity. This can affect the workplace significantly.

In the first weeks after one's symptoms appear, it can be awkward if the illness is unknown or is being hidden for fear of stigma and judgment. It's not like people coming to work while undergoing chemotherapy treatments for cancer; in that case, they would likely feel comfortable disclosing the illness and creating a plan to work around it as best they could. Therefore, with a physical illness, there would be zero stigma; people would have a much clearer idea of what to say and how to act around the person dealing with it.

That isn't the case with mental illness. And that's how one in four is really four in four. Mental illness touches us all. The following helps us to visualize this concept:

Figure 1 represents a group of one hundred people in a work-place. It could represent an entire company or a department within a company. (For emphasis, I have chosen to represent the more conservative estimate of mental illness affecting one in five people, which is the absolute minimum.)

Figure 1

THE IMPACT OF WORKPLACE MENTAL ILLNESS

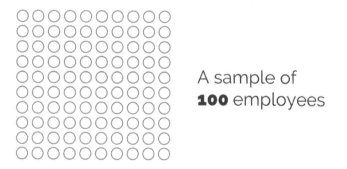

A sample of **100** employees

Figure 2 shows a random set of individuals suffering from a mental illness at a ratio of one in five.

Figure 2

THE IMPACT OF WORKPLACE MENTAL ILLNESS

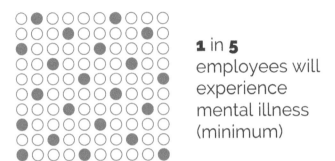

1 in **5** employees will experience mental illness (minimum)

Figure 3 shows how one person with symptoms of a mental illness affects those in their immediate sphere—their team members, their direct reports and their managers.

Figure 3

THE IMPACT OF WORKPLACE MENTAL ILLNESS

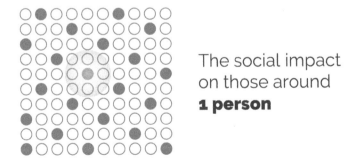

The social impact on those around **1 person**

Figure 4 shows the residual effect caused by all of those with mental illness on the people around them. It indicates that *every single* person in this community of one hundred is affected by mental illness.

Figure 4

THE IMPACT OF WORKPLACE MENTAL ILLNESS

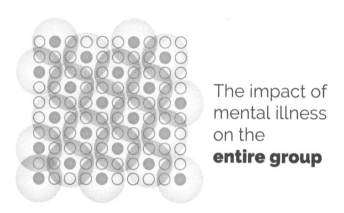

The impact of mental illness on the **entire group**

These images clearly illustrate why mental illness cannot be ignored or swept aside as it often has been by leaders of corporations. Mental illness is a very real obstacle for every organization— one that is draining resources, reducing productivity, and causing losses in profit.

While mental illness cannot be eradicated, the challenge it poses can be managed much better than it is currently. A core cause of mismanaging mental illness in corporate environments is the stigma that still surrounds it. But this difficult and delicate topic can be addressed and improved upon.

Consider this: if stigma is not addressed and dramatically reduced, all other educational and support programs will never have a lasting impact.

THE LEAST MOODY MAN
IN THE WORLD

For many years after my heart surgery, I enjoyed the kind of health we can easily take for granted. In fact, I *intentionally* took it for granted. It seemed to me I had faced my big health challenge when I was young, and a fair reward would be a life of stable health. For a long while, that was exactly true. I didn't think about my health or how my body was working unless I had a cold or a flu, or unless I was working out. It felt gloriously free.

I finished elementary school without any more heart problems, and I was cleared after my five-year check-up while in high school. My heart function was officially normal, and I didn't need to worry about it ever again, nor did I need to limit my activities in any way.

Thinking like a normal boy again, my focus shifted from serious stuff, like how my heart was functioning, to the more important matters: girls, music, and dirt bikes. During this time, one of the greatest gifts my mom gave me was teaching me the importance of being romantic.

She noticed I had a crush on one of my classmates in grade seven. One day, I mentioned I was worried about the boys teasing me if all I wanted to do was hang out and talk with her. Mom's response had a massive impact on me.

She said, "Don't question yourself; you are thinking the right way. If you like a girl, then it's the girl's opinion that matters, not the boys' … girls love boys who are romantic and thoughtful like you are, so don't change. The boys will like you and be your friend regardless."

In that one moment, my mom solidified an instinct she saw in me, and I've been a hopeless romantic ever since. What a great gift.

I went through high school like any other teen. My main concerns were my friends, my girlfriend, my academics, and my hobbies. I was a good student, had great friends, and spent most of those years in a long-term relationship with my high school sweetheart. Life brought challenges, but overall, it was a positive and healthy time in my life.

By the time I went to the University of Waterloo to study theater and speech communication, my main personality traits had long been established. I was happy-go-lucky, friendly, sociable, fun-loving, optimistic, positive, supportive, and eager to please. Most people in my life described me as an all-around nice guy who was always in a good mood. While some of this reflected exactly who I was, a significant part came as a result of my heart defect and surgery experience.

The simple truth is this: it's easy to be in a good mood when you feel constant gratitude for being alive and healthy. I never forgot how lucky I was to recover from my heart defect, and I never lost my sense of gratitude for every moment I was given.

My Dad's Message

My dad was a real estate agent in Orillia, Ontario, for much of his career, and on a certain day when I was in grade four, I was with him when he had to stop at his office. We parked beside the building, which had on one wall a large mural that honored Stephen Leacock, a famous writer and professor at McGill University in Montreal, Quebec, who kept a summer home in Orillia. The mural showed Professor Leacock holding his hat and scratching his head. The accompanying quotation read: "I am a firm believer in luck. But I find the harder I work, the luckier I get."

My dad took a moment to make sure I had seen the mural and read the quotation, then he said, "Son, that is the truth. If you always work hard and never quit, you will have more than your fair share of luck in your life."

That message took hold of me in every way. I loved the idea behind it. I watched the truth of it in my dad and how he lived his life, and I believed it. What a wonderful message from my father. It has served me well in everything I share in this book, and it continues to serve me to this day.

My dad has always been an incredibly important part of my life—a father, a mentor, a best friend, a zero-interest bank (on more than one occasion!), a shoulder to cry on, and a guide. I could write an entire other book just on the ways he has influenced me for the better.

Being Nice with No Agenda

Being a happy-go-lucky, all-around nice guy did create an interesting situation during my years at the University of Waterloo, in Ontario. This trait caused me to learn something interesting about how many others see the world.

Early in my first year, I attended a play created specifically for frosh students. It covered many serious topics such as sexual harassment by a teacher, homosexuality, fear of judgment and peer pressure, drug and alcohol abuse, and more. The play was so well written and performed, I stayed after the production to compliment the actors and director. I didn't think any more of it, and after saying a few nice words to them, I went on my way.

Almost two years later, I was fully engaged in the theater program and was in the midst of rehearsals for a mainstage production of *The Crucible*, directed by the very same director. In fact, some of the actors from that frosh play were in this production, and I had become friends with almost everyone in the program. (This tends to happen in theater, given the time spent together in such intimate settings.)

After one particular rehearsal, we went out together, feeling relaxed, and enjoyed a few drinks. Out of nowhere, the director said to me, "I get it! I finally understand you. You actually *are* this genuine and nice!"

"Thanks, but what do you mean? What made you say that?" I replied, totally confused.

"When I first met you," she replied, "you introduced yourself and complimented my frosh play. I thought you were just being political and kissing up to a director who might cast you one day, so I didn't trust you. But now that I've gotten to know you, I see you actually *mean* all the nice things you say—and that you don't have an agenda."

This admission blew my mind. I couldn't believe she'd thought that about me initially, but I especially couldn't believe it took almost two years of consistent behavior on my part before she fully trusted me and believed I was genuinely nice. In fact, for a while afterward, I was upset that others' cynicism would create doubt about my sincerity. Eventually, though, I realized I couldn't control the thoughts and feelings of other people. My best option was always to be myself. If I was "too nice" for others, they would figure it out eventually.

Jumping out of a Perfectly Good Airplane

Although I had always enjoyed heights and speed, such as flying, fast cars, and roller coasters, I remember the first time I thought, "I'd like to try jumping out of planes." That happened at age seventeen when I was watching *Point Break*, a movie starring Patrick Swayze and Keanu Reeves, which includes a dramatic skydiving sequence. Later, I learned that many of the technical details from that sequence didn't match reality, such as the length of the skydive (at four minutes, it was nearly twice as long as the highest altitude jump recreational skydivers would make) and their ability to speak to each other during freefall (even if you yell as loud as you can, the sound won't make it to each other's ears). Still, it fully captured the beauty of the sport. I knew immediately I'd try skydiving as soon as I was nineteen and could legally do it.

As my nineteenth birthday approached, I organized a large group that included my oldest brother, my girlfriend, and several friends—eleven in all. We signed up to take the course and complete our first skydive together. That initial jump was terrifying, thrilling, and magical all at once. I knew before my feet touched the ground that I had to do it again.

I was the only one out of our group who took up the sport seriously. My brother jumped eight times—including on the morning of his wedding day—while a few others jumped two or three times, but several only jumped that one time. I went on to amass 168 skydives and obtain my "C" license from the Canadian Sport Parachute Association.

Although 168 jumps may seem like a great number of skydives to someone who has never jumped, it's an incredibly small number in the world of serious skydivers. Many regular skydivers have logged between five hundred and two thousand jumps, while some instructors, tandem masters, and competitive skydivers have ten thousand or more skydives under their belts. Turning to a golf analogy, I'd be called an above-average player with a single-digit handicap, while these pros are playing on the PGA Tour.

Despite this comparison, I had remarkable experiences along the way, including a night skydive. What an absolute thrill to jump out of a Twin Otter aircraft into the darkness at six thousand feet over Florida, with the sky above full of stars and a full moon, and below the ground was a patchwork of street and city lights. Floating down was an experience I will never forget. To find the drop zone, I looked for cars that were lined up facing the landing area, beaming their headlights. The drop zone was actually easy to see due to this unusual light formation. That night, I was able to land as softly as I did in the light of day.

Another highlight was a high-altitude skydive from twenty-two thousand feet that included an incredible two-minute-and-ten-second freefall, when an average freefall lasted from forty-five to sixty seconds to just over a minute. Also in Florida, when it was thirty-three degrees Celsius and muggy on the ground, the temperature was a brisk zero degrees Celsius when we exited the King Air (a plane once used as an executive aircraft before small jets were available)! To have a sense of how long the freefall was on that skydive, sit and stare at a stopwatch for two minutes and ten seconds. Visualize me falling that entire time—and then I pulled my parachute and began a four-minute descent. It was awesome.

Finally, I had the opportunity to take part in a large formation skydive with twenty-three people in total. My average jumps were with one to four others; only on a few occasions was I part of formations with seven to ten. Being in the air in freefall with twenty-two other people and successfully making a pre-designed formation before separating for the parachute descent was a challenge and a thrill.

Why I Stopped Skydiving

By the time I stopped skydiving, I had logged more than one and a half hours in freefall. That statistic makes me smile. Today, I can say I've spent one and a half hours of my life falling at 120 miles per hour!

My roommate during my first year of university, who quickly became a dear friend, asked if I would continue skydiving once I got married. The question confused me; skydiving was an important part of my life, and I had no intention of stopping.

I asked him, "What does being married have to do with it?"

Always a man of few but very well-thought-out words, he replied, "Just seems like a dick way to die."

I was irritated with him and completely disagreed. Yes, there were inherent risks in skydiving, but I took it seriously and had an extremely conservative approach to the sport. For me, risk wasn't an issue, so I ignored his comment and forgot about it.

Several years later, in July 2007, while engaged to my now wife Anna, I took her skydiving just outside of Montreal. She completed a tandem jump while I jumped solo out of the same plane. We met on the ground, still buzzing from the adrenaline high, and celebrated the experience with a kiss. At that moment, I thought Anna would want to take up the sport and we might become a skydiving couple.

But life took over. It was the last time either of us went skydiving.

Anna and I married in February 2008. That spring, I began thinking of skydiving again, as I had done every spring for fourteen years. But this time, something was different. This time, I was married to Anna, and a voice in my head kept saying my wise friend's words: "Seems like a dick way to die."

Like in the Chris Nolan film *Inception* starring Leonardo DiCaprio, my friend had managed to plant a powerful idea deep in my mind. A few years after he said it, I realized he was right. I had to stop skydiving. I just couldn't risk doing that to Anna.

While the chances are low, if something goes wrong during a skydive, the potential for injury or death is very real. If I suffered a serious injury or died doing it and left Anna to pick up the pieces, what a selfish act that would be.

I look back fondly at my skydiving years with gratitude that my health—especially my surgically repaired heart—allowed me to "fly" in that way. I don't explicitly believe in reincarnation; however, if I did have a past life, I must have been a bird. I don't only enjoy flying—I'm in a place of total peace while doing it. I have many vivid memories of freefalling, an intense and surreal experience of using my body to literally fly as I fall, followed by parachute descents that are beautifully serene.

During each parachute flight, it's normal for skydivers to look down past their dangling feet at the ground several thousand feet below. One time when I did this, I saw an eagle about a hundred feet below me. It struck me that it was the first (and still only) time I'd ever seen the top of a bird soaring in flight. I followed this majestic bird for a while, moving at almost the same speed. It was magical.

THE MOST IMPORTANT
LEAP OF MY LIFE

After I graduated from university in 1998 with a Bachelor of Arts in Theater and Speech Communication, I spent my early career working in sales in Toronto. Although being a salesperson wasn't a good fit for me, I continued to be healthy and happy overall. My dislike of my work and, in part, living in the greater Toronto area led me to follow my girlfriend to Montreal. She had moved there to attend McGill University, and while visiting her each month, I fell in love with the city. Despite my inability to speak French, I decided to move there too and find a new career path. While this could have, and maybe should have, been a scary and uncertain time, I found it fun and exciting to take the leap into a new adventure.

Soon after moving in with my girlfriend and settling into our beautiful apartment near Mount Royal Park, the largest park at the center Montreal, the reality of finding a job in an unknown and primarily French-speaking city hit me. *This wouldn't be easy.*

I spent several months working at my Ontario job remotely while I looked for something local. I was selling Registered Education Savings Plans (RESPs), which was similar to being an insurance agent. From Montreal, I'd set up a string of appointments in the Toronto area, then go there for a few days at a time. This arrangement paid the bills but wasn't workable long term.

One afternoon a few months after moving, my girlfriend and I had a drink with friends in the Thompson House, McGill's graduate house. One of her new friends was also taking her Master of Arts in English. This young woman studied part-time and worked part-time for McGill University in Development and Alumni Relations. During this fateful meeting, she asked me about my background, skills, and interests. It struck her that I would be a perfect fit for the work she was doing.

When I learned more about the nature of fundraising for a university, I completely agreed.

She was kind enough to take my résumé and pass it on to the HR people at McGill. Before long, I was being interviewed, and I ultimately secured a position in the Development and Alumni Relations Office of the Faculty of Engineering. It was by far the most interesting and engaging job I'd ever had, and I was thrilled to start a new career. I loved my work and my colleagues, and simultaneously my relationship with my girlfriend deepened. Before long, I planned to propose.

But then, for the second time, my life changed radically for me because of an illness that appeared out of nowhere and for no apparent reason.

DEPRESSION HITS

The first symptoms of mental illness I experienced came in the form of mild depression, which lasted for two months. It was early 2002, I was twenty-six years old, and my fourteen-year run of excellent health had come to a screeching halt.

I had no idea what depression was at the time, and I didn't even consider mental illness as a potential cause for my symptoms. Not only was I happy-go-lucky and a contender for the least moody man around, but my life was going exceptionally well. There was simply no reason for me to feel down, let alone depressed, so I assumed I had some sort of strange flu.

Depression, also known as clinical depression or major depressive disorder, is defined by the Canadian Mental Health Association (CMHA) as a "common and serious medical illness that negatively affects how you feel, the way you think and how you act." (See Glossary of terms at end of this book for the definitions of more key terms.)

This definition held true for me, as the symptoms I experienced included decreased physical and mental energy, a slight ache in my entire body, a sense that every movement and thought took more energy than normal, and a need for extra sleep and rest. Given that this came on suddenly in January 2002 and lasted two months, it was reasonable to assume I had caught a persistent bug, so I waited it out.

Describing clinical depression is an interesting challenge, considering the word "depressed" is often used to name a short-lived mood such as sadness or melancholy. This can cause people to think depression is something we have a measure of control over. However, for me, clinical depression is closer to the worst flu I'd ever had than any emotional sadness. It's incredibly physical; I can feel it in every fiber of my being. For many, clinical depression does include emotional sadness as the main symptom, but for others (me included), clinical depression doesn't bring sadness, but rather causes feelings of being shut off from everyone. When it was severe, I was unable to function normally and slept many extra hours a day.

A Prisoner in a Plexiglass Box

One way I describe depression is this: You feel like you have been imprisoned in a plexiglass box. You can go through life seeing everything and everyone around you, but you can't touch, or feel, or smell, or taste anything. You are numb. Your energy (both physical and mental) can be lower than you've ever experienced.

For me, being clinically depressed is like being a non-person, totally robbed of the simple things that make life wonderful, like energy, mental acuity, and the ability to connect with those around me in meaningful ways. If someone tells you they are clinically depressed, I implore you to first feel empathy, because that person is suffering in a profound way.

All of these challenges are amplified when depression becomes more extreme, moving from mild to moderate and then severe. While my first depressive episode through January and February of 2002 was mild, my next one was moderate and carried more powerful symptoms. That episode lasted from July to September of 2003. Throughout this two-month period, I felt everything I just described only more intensely, and it was affecting my ability to work. Certainly the quality of my work and my life were noticeably suffering.

I forced myself to work through my first several depressive episodes, mainly because I had no idea what was happening. I later realized I was falling prey to self-stigma—that is, my negative thoughts towards, and fear of, mental illness caused me to refuse to even consider that I might be suffering from a mental illness (more on that topic in the coming chapters). But I couldn't deny that putting in a full day at work went from enjoyable—I loved my job and felt lucky to have it—to challenging, to extremely difficult, and eventually to impossible.

For example, I found myself taking bathroom breaks every thirty to forty-five minutes, just so I could be alone. I needed separation from the people I had to talk with and the work I had to do. Activities that used to be easy seemed impossible. I would sometimes spend twenty minutes in the bathroom, staring at myself in the mirror and wondering how I could get through the day. It was terrifying to suddenly be robbed of many of my social skills, which were fundamental to who I was as a person and an employee.

Lunchtime also became a challenge. I worked in downtown Montreal, so going out to eat was common. However, I started going out alone— to get away from people with whom I normally loved spending time— and walking St. Catherine Street, trying to decide where to eat. More often than not, I would waste my entire lunch hour wandering back and forth, unable to select a place. Something as simple as making a choice of where to eat lunch suddenly became difficult. To this day, I vividly remember those indecisive walks, mostly because I felt so lost and alone.

My First Severe Depression

In January and February of 2004, I experienced my first severe depressive episode. Although I took some vacation time and several sick days, I tried to do my job through the rest of this episode. I honestly have no idea how I managed. I had never felt anything like this in my entire life; my body was in constant dull pain, my mind seemed sedated, and my energy levels were nil from the moment I woke up.

Everything, even things I normally found easy, like casual conversation and writing emails, suddenly became Herculean tasks. Despite putting in my best efforts, it was evident to people at work that something was wrong. I wasn't even remotely the same person I once was at the office; my normally cheerful and friendly personality had suddenly vanished, and my productivity suffered. My boss was clearly concerned and asked if I was okay several times a week. No one knew what to do or say, including me.

CREATE YOUR
STIGMAZERO WORKPLACE
PART 2

Mental Illness vs. Physical Illness: A Manner of Speaking

There's a key difference in the way we speak about major physical illnesses, such as a heart defect and cancer, versus mental illnesses. And that key difference always comes down to understanding, knowledge, and awareness—and how a lack thereof can create fear and stigma.

We're set up to have an overdeveloped vocabulary of negative, stigma-filled words regarding mental illness. They appear in the movies and television shows we watch, and have done so for years. As a way to illustrate this, I employ this exercise in the programs within The StigmaZero Online Training Academy.

First, I ask a simple (if loaded) question:

> Please write down the first negative, stigma-filled, judgmental word that comes to mind regarding mental illnesses such as depression, anxiety, bipolar disorder, and so on.

As you can imagine, people hesitate at first. But after reassuring them we're in a safe space, I offer the first word and the ice quickly breaks.

"Crazy," I say, to lead things off.

The following list shows the most common words that arise when people do this exercise.

Abnormal	Fruitcake	Nutter	Simpleton
Abusive	Half-wit	Odd	Spastic
Bonkers	Head case	Oddball	Spaz
Brain damaged	Helpless	Off their rocker	Straightjacket
Brain-dead	Hypochondriac	Out of it	Strange
Breakdown	Idiot	Padded cells	Thick
Childish	Insane	Paranoid	Troubled
Confused	Intimidating	Perverted	Unpredictable
Crazy	Irrational	Pill popper	Unreliable
Deformed	Lazy	Problem	Unstable
Demented	Loony	Psycho	Veg
Disturbed	Loser	Reject	Vegetable
Downy	Mad	Retard	Violent
Drugged-up	Mental	Sad	Wacky
Dumb	Not all there	Scary	Weak
Embarrassing	Nut-bar	Schizo	Weird
Empty	Nutcase	Screw loose	Weirdo
Freak	Nuts	Sick in the head	White coats

After the initial discomfort of considering these objectionable words, the floodgates open and the labels come fast and easy. We may not use these words, but we've heard them, some of them countless times. We have easy access to them. We know them.

My point is driven home by the second part of this exercise, when I ask them to do the same thing, but with a twist:

Please write down negative, stigma-filled, judgmental words—but this time describing cancer.

Silence. Blank stares.

Often, someone will be clever and comment about lung cancer caused by smoking. There may be judgments about that. In these cases, I ask them to complete the exercise while considering cancers unrelated to lifestyle or behavior, such as breast cancer or colon cancer.

Silence. Blank stares.

And then what follows is a dawning realization of why they can't come up with a single word. It's because in today's society, we don't see, hear, or use stigma-filled words regarding cancer or any illness understood to be *something that happens to* a person. We feel empathy for individuals who've had the misfortune to be diagnosed with any illness deemed not their fault. And when we feel empathy, we don't feel stigma.

A DARK WALK DOWN MEMORY LANE

As my depressive episodes kept returning and became increasingly more severe, I was forced to face the reality that something was wrong with me. However, I was still under the influence of a major self-stigma regarding mental illness. I denied having a mental illness of any kind, and I flat-out refused the notion that I may need medical treatment.

When these two opposing forces came to a head, I had to admit that something was needed beyond waiting and hoping. So I came up with the idea of seeing a psychologist.

For many people, this strategy works well. Commonly, the onset of a mental illness is caused by a complex set of factors, including stress, unresolved emotional trauma, and more. But for me, my motivation was one of pure avoidance and procrastination. I'm struck by the irony of my decision to see a psychologist. As a healthy, happy, twenty-six-year-old man who was experiencing depression with no apparent cause, I chose a lengthy process of talk therapy in the hopes of finding something from my past that could be the trigger. I made this choice almost entirely to avoid seeing a medical doctor who might refer me to a psychiatrist, who might then diagnose me with a mental illness and prescribe a treatment.

There was only one reason for my actions: the powerful self-stigma I was suffering.

Instead of seeing diagnosis and treatment as positive steps on the road to recovery, I was terrified and willing to do almost anything to avoid that path. It would take me another eighteen months to learn this lesson, but my actions during that time helped me understand the formidable power that stigma and self-stigma have on behavior when it comes to mental illness.

My experience of having had a heart defect and major surgery would ultimately provide me with the context to see this truth: we don't behave this way with illnesses we understand. But that realization came much later.

In the following pages, I share the traumatic experiences I discussed with my psychologist over several sessions and describe her determination at the end of my last session with her.

Mom's Mis-scheduled Suicide Attempt

It was Saturday morning. I was sitting at the kitchen table, finishing my lunch and playing with my toy cars (my favorite was a red Porsche). I didn't have a care in the world, although that was more because I was only eight years old and not because everything was fine at home. In fact, my parents had divorced a few months prior, and Mom didn't seem happy at all.

My two older brothers were doing their own thing too, and the mood that morning was relaxed. Around noon, my oldest brother, who was eighteen at the time, noticed that Mom was still not up. While it was normal for her to sleep quite late, sleeping until noon was unusual. Besides, her friend was scheduled to arrive shortly with her kids for a visit. It was time to wake Mom up so she could get ready.

"Let me come with you!" I said to my brother when he went upstairs to awaken her. As we walked down the hall to her door, which was closed, I had no idea something terrifying and awful was about to happen. Until then, it seemed like a normal Saturday.

My brother opened the bedroom door. Mom was lying on her back, and I caught a glimpse of something yellow by her mouth. Before I could make out any details, however, my brother's hand covered my face. In a gesture for which I have felt immense gratitude, he saved me from really seeing Mom in this state. Given how she looked, he thought she may actually be dead. I'm amazed that he had the presence of mind to protect his little brother from that sight.

"Go downstairs now and call Nancy!" he ordered. By the tone of his voice, I knew this was serious and I should do exactly as I was told. Nancy, our next-door neighbor, was a registered nurse.

I ran downstairs, called Nancy, and told her something was wrong with Mom. I told her to come right away. Nancy understood the seriousness immediately. She didn't ask for more information; she hung up and arrived at our front door moments later. Her quick reaction may well have saved Mom's life that day.

My memories of what happened next are like a movie montage set to music. Multiple things flashed by my eyes, and I could see each one in vivid detail, but the overall picture was sped up and condensed. Here's how the movie unfolded.

Nancy arriving, looking concerned but not panicked.
Nancy rushing upstairs and returning very quickly, looking
panicked and a little sick.
Nancy calling the ambulance, then trying to keep my brothers
and me calm.
Mom's friend arriving with her kids. Based on my brother's and
Nancy's reaction, it was the worst possible time.
Everyone feeling upset and Mom's friend crying.
Mom's friend's son and I playing with my cars at the kitchen
table as the paramedics arrived.
The paramedics carrying an empty stretcher upstairs.
The paramedics carrying the stretcher with Mom on it back
downstairs. I had never seen her so sick; her skin looked gray.

At some point, Dad arrived. He had been living at the family cottage since their divorce. We were living with him and would visit Mom on some weekends, like we had this one. I could feel the stress and tension in the house, but I didn't really understand what had happened.

It would be years before I knew and understood the full story of that day. Once I was old enough, Mom spoke openly about why she had tried to take her own life. Leading up to that day and following the divorce, she had been in one of the worst depressions of her life, and she'd never had success with antidepressants. Mom had also been an alcoholic for years, so she often self-medicated instead of, or in addition to, her treatments.

It turns out she had been planning her suicide for some time. Had her actions gone according to plan, she would have died without question. She never meant to do it while her boys were there, nor when her friend was coming to visit. In fact, she planned to do it the following weekend when she'd be alone. But on this Friday, with her three sons in the house, she became confused after drinking late into the night. This caused her to get her weekends mixed up. Thinking she was alone in the house, she took ninety sleeping pills.

Perhaps it was a subconscious cry for help to attempt suicide with people in the house rather than when she was alone. Perhaps it was nothing more than pure coincidence. Regardless, this change in weekends saved her life.

With Nancy's help, she arrived at the hospital just in time and, after a week in a coma, she made a miraculous recovery. I was told that her case was studied at the Newmarket hospital, because it didn't make any medical sense that she survived.

The doctor who cared for her during her recovery told my dad, "For a woman who tried to end her life, she sure is fighting to live. I have never seen anyone fight this hard."

As it turned out, my mom would live for another twenty-three years before succumbing to cancer. For twenty of those years, I lived with the belief that what Mom had done was weak, cowardly, and selfish. It was something to forgive her for, which I tried hard to do. Yet I felt hurt and angry that she would even consider doing such a thing, let alone actually go through with it, and a part of me reserved judgment on her actions.

I am ashamed of my lack of empathy and understanding. I am also ashamed that I had such a strong stigma clouding my judgment and preventing me from seeing the truth.

I first began to understand this event when I experienced clinical depression firsthand. My longest depressive episode was three months and one week. I can honestly say I never considered suicide—in large part because I had such a strong anti-suicide stance, given what Mom had done. At that time, I believed I'd never do that to my loved ones; I thought I was better than that.

While I may have come by that opinion honestly, I would later see it as shameful. Who was I to judge another person's suffering? Besides, what would I feel and do if my depressive episodes lasted six months? A year? Two years? While at the bottom of my deepest and longest depression, I realized how it's possible for people to be broken down by mental illness to the point where they believe their only way out is suicide.

Suicide isn't about weakness or selfishness. It is about suffering. And we can only help those who experience suicidal thoughts through our empathy, understanding, support, and love. Our judgment doesn't belong.

One of the greatest gifts of my life was learning this lesson before my mom passed. I had the opportunity to apologize to her for my years of quiet judgment, and for my lack of empathy and understanding. I told her I now understood that, on the day she tried to take her life, she wasn't trying to hurt us. Rather, she intended to end her pain in the only way she knew how at that moment.

Mom was kind enough to forgive me. She explained that after years of untreated depression and self-medicating with alcohol and prescription sleeping aids, she had lost any sense of a way out of her situation. She had come to a dark and despairing place where she believed she only had one choice that would end the pain. Better treatments and more social support would have likely helped her had there been less stigma. As a result, Mom might have never reached that dark place of despair. In fact, her terrible experience with mental illness, including the stigma she faced and the lack of treatment options and support, largely inspired me to dedicate my life to ending mental illness stigma. That would ultimately lead me to start StigmaZero, and write this book.

But as often happens with individuals who suffer from mental illness and addiction, my mom's experience was complicated. Although she was able to recover in many ways, she never totally stopped drinking. Her relationship with alcohol was a contentious issue between the two of us as well as between her and the rest of our family. (I share one of the ways her relationship with alcohol affected me in a later chapter.)

Author's Note: I seriously considered not including this story about my mom's attempted suicide in this book. It's more her story than mine, and I didn't want to exploit her in any way. The more I considered it, though, the more I realized that the reasons not to include this story were rooted in stigma and my fear of judgment that readers might feel towards her. That's when I knew it had to be included—not only because it was a part of my experience, but because my goal is to fight stigma. The only way to do that is for me to speak openly and share with you and the world—even the most difficult parts.

Did I Have Thoughts of Suicide?

"Have you ever attempted or considered suicide?"

In many social contexts, that question would be unusual or inappropriate. However, it is one of the most common questions I'm asked during my keynote lectures or workshops. And it should be. My audiences have just heard stories about how mental illness affected my life through several three-month-long depressive episodes.

"No, fortunately I never went to thoughts of suicide" is always my answer, which is true. Not for one second did I consider ending my life, even during my most severely depressed times. That is not a comment on my strength, character, mental fortitude, or even desire to live. Nor is it a judgment on those who suffer terribly for so long that they believe there's no other choice.

Rather, in part, it's because I formed a deep-seated opinion about suicide when I was eight years old because of my mom's attempt. Also, my severe depressive episodes lasted only a few months rather than years. And, I believe, I found a way to break free of stigma and the loneliness and despair that comes with mental illness.

It is important to understand, however, that not all clinical depression leads to suicidal thoughts or actions. Confusion on this point is due to people thinking that if they suffered from a moderate clinical depression for years, they don't have a mental illness or "real depression" because they haven't had suicidal thoughts. That is simply not true.

Like me, many people experience clinical depression of varying degrees of severity without suicidal thoughts. Let me emphasize this: *Depression is a serious illness that significantly affects an individual's quality of life, and it should be treated as soon as possible.* As I stated in the disclaimer at the start of this book, if you are reading this and experiencing suicidal thoughts, please know these two truths: **you have value, and there is help available**. Please search for crisis, help, or suicide hotlines in your area.

NOT AN AVERAGE GRADE SCHOOL EXPERIENCE

Another difficult period in my life I shared with the psychologist included the two years I spent in grades seven and eight in Scarborough, Ontario, a suburb on the east end of Toronto. I lived there during my last two years of elementary school. In fact, those were the last two years I lived in the Toronto area with my mom before moving to Orillia, Ontario, to live with my dad.

Although I made many lifelong friends during those two years, terrible things that I'll never forget also happened. First, as described earlier, I had my open-heart surgery in the latter part of grade seven. That alone made those two years challenging and remarkable. In addition, my classmates and I had to deal with a very unusual teacher we called Mr. O.

In grade seven, I would have emphatically said Mr. O. was a great teacher. He found interesting ways to challenge me to learn new things, and he seemed passionate about teaching. However, he changed dramatically in grade eight, when he seemed to grow bitter and controlling. He said and did things that would hurt his students' feelings and negatively affect our confidence. He said to me and others that we "wouldn't amount to anything." What a terrible experience to have a teacher inspire us and build our confidence, only to knock it down soon after.

In 2017, I attended a reunion of our grade eight graduating class. There, many of us spent time darkly reminiscing all the mean, bizarre, and distasteful things Mr. O. said to some of us. While he never physically abused anyone, what he did amounted to psychological abuse.

We never found out why Mr. O. changed between grade seven and grade eight. It seemed that as long as we behaved and didn't question his unorthodox teaching methods, he was fairly pleasant. However, as we matured and started to resist, or when personal problems in students' lives created distractions from schoolwork, he became resentful, bitter, and mean. He continued to teach for many years, although happiness seemed to elude him. At the reunion, one of our classmates mentioned often seeing him drinking alone at a Scarborough restaurant and bar.

Raymond

In addition to dealing with Mr. O., we were faced with a tragedy. One of our classmates, a dynamic and popular boy named Raymond, was diagnosed with leukemia. None of us could believe that would happen to Raymond, who was a healthy, energetic, and vital young man. At first, we all felt certain he'd be able to fight the leukemia and recover. Unfortunately, the illness quickly overwhelmed him, and he succumbed within only a few months.

How could this happen? His passing shocked our class, tearing a hole right through us. None of us will ever forget the day we found out he had died, nor will we forget Raymond. My most vivid memories include opening my front door that morning to find my dear friend, Raymond's girlfriend, Clara, in tears on my doorstep. I was in shock and disbelief when she told me Raymond was gone.

At school that day, we gathered in our classroom before going to the church for a scheduled rehearsal of our upcoming confirmation (our school was Catholic). Then, after all of the sadness and weirdness of rehearsing a ceremony while in the immediate stages of grief, while walking back to our school, several of us broke into a run. The route from the church to the school took us along a street called Military Trail, which had a ravine and woods on each side. We bolted down one of the paths, running and screaming in pain, anger, and confusion.

I'll never forget that raw, emotional moment.

Altar Boys

Unbelievably, we had one more major challenge to face. Since our school was Catholic, it was affiliated with a local church. Several male students, including me, my best friend Marc, our friend Anthony, and a few others volunteered to be altar boys for some of the masses. To be honest, many of us were only interested because it meant time outside the classroom!

At first, the experience was positive; we helped Father run mass and had fun being away from class. Of those who volunteered, the majority were quite outgoing and had strong personalities, including me. Two of our classmates who volunteered, however, were quiet and shy. At the time, we couldn't know that Father targeted those two boys, ultimately sexually abusing them both. When it was announced that Father was charged with abusing two of our classmates, we were in shock. None of us believed he was even capable of such a terrible thing. How could I have looked up to him and thought him a good person? It was heartbreaking to learn about people and the nature of evil in this way.

THE LEAST IN NEED

My time with the psychologist ended abruptly after six sessions. We had discussed my past emotional traumas, and it was the psychologist, not me, who ended the therapy. In doing so, she offered me an incredibly kind gesture that would prove a major turning point in my fight against stigma.

She said, "Jason, I have listened to you share the many traumas and challenges you have faced in your life, and I have something important to tell you. I have seventy-eight patients, and you are, by far, the least in need of my services. You're one of the most emotionally organized people I've ever met, and your depressions are not due to anything in your past."

I was stunned by this statement. She was helping me see that all the traumas I had experienced due to my mom's attempted suicide and the many challenges I faced in grades seven and eight were not connected to the onset of mental illness I was facing in my late twenties. What an important revelation for me!

She continued, "I'm not a psychiatrist, so I cannot offer a diagnosis of a mental illness or prescribe treatment, but my professional opinion is that you have bipolar disorder. It's not a condition you can address through talk therapy alone, especially when your emotional state is so sound."

"So what do I do then?" I asked.

"See a psychiatrist and share what I've told you. If you need to, go to the emergency ward of the hospital. There, they will likely prescribe treatment, and if they do, take it. This isn't your fault; it's an illness."

And with that, she wished me good luck. I never saw her again, but her parting gift changed my life in more ways than I could imagine. Although I'd heard the same essential message (that what I was dealing with was an illness and it wasn't my fault) from my fiancée for the past two years, something clicked when the psychologist said it to me.

The Right Message at the Right Time

Here was a medical professional who, after months of talk therapy, was telling me I was wasting my time continuing down that path. This became the right message at the right time from the right person, and I finally heard it. I knew then that my biggest barrier was not my illness but the stigma surrounding it—and the fear and paralysis it caused.

In that moment, I finally decided to break down the self-stigma and start thinking of this new challenge as what it was—an illness no different than my heart defect. One of my first acts was understanding what bipolar is, which began a lifetime of research into mental illness and stigma. The definition from the National Institute of Mental Health is: "Bipolar disorder, also known as manic-depressive illness, is a brain disorder that causes unusual shifts in mood, energy, activity levels, and the ability to carry out day-to-day tasks. Episodes of depression with mixed features (having depression and manic symptoms at the same time) are also possible."

It was clear I would have a hard road ahead, but I had finally conquered the worst and most difficult challenge of having a mental illness. I was finally becoming free of stigma and self-stigma—and that has saved my life.

CREATE YOUR
STIGMAZERO WORKPLACE
PART 3

My Issue with the Word "Issue"

As a person who has faced the challenges of both open-heart surgery and bipolar disorder, I'm all too familiar with the kind of language people use to describe illness. It ranges from clinical and benign to negative and charged with a discriminatory attitude. Let me explain my issue with the use of the word "issue" when speaking of mental illness.

Of the many definitions of this word, two of them apply to this argument:

- a personal or emotional problem

Example: I had issues that prevented me from doing well in school.

- any problem or difficulty

Example: Sorry I'm late—I had an issue with parking.

I fully acknowledge that many people who currently use the word "issue" when describing a mental illness (for example, "Dave is having issues with depression") do so with no negative intent or stigma. I also recognize that, based on the definition of issue as "any problem or difficulty," using it to describe a mental illness is, indeed, a correct use of the word.

However, I would argue that there's an inherent, underlying judgment, deriving from the existence of stigma in this use of "issue."

It's based on one simple distinction: People don't say, "Steve has an issue with his heart," or "Marc is in the hospital due to issues with cancer," or "Anna has cellular health issues."

In these contexts, most people understand "issue" to mean the first definition, namely "a personal or emotional problem." And we intrinsically understand that, using these examples, a heart problem or cancer are by no means personal or emotional problems.

Mental illness, on the other hand, is commonly lumped into this category. Why? Because many people—even those who are empathetic and well-intentioned—don't understand the various mental illnesses well enough to know that they aren't personal or emotional problems.

This lack of knowledge can create fear, stigma, and discrimination, even if only on a subconscious level. Thus, the use of the word "issue" carries a subtle but powerful effect.

It's best to understand mental illness as a clinical—and highly physical—illness with wide-ranging symptoms that can't be changed by sorting out a personal or emotional problem. I tried for two years to fight through the symptoms of bipolar disorder without any treatment. Doing so was as wasteful and unsuccessful as trying to meditate my way to a healthy heart.

Now hear the difference. These horrible, life-altering symptoms of mental illness are being described as an "issue," while a person's virus is called an "illness." Sometimes the subtlest (and often unintentional) forms of stigma in our language can be the most hurtful and difficult to change.

If you want to stop the negative use of the word "issue," adopt this simple but effective trick: before saying or writing anything about someone with a mental illness, ask if you would use the same language if he or she had cancer.

SHEDDING SELF-STIGMA

In March 2004, I came out of the severe depressive episode that began in January of that year, only to experience another in July and August. For the second summer in a row, I was overwhelmed by the symptoms of clinical depression. This was especially frustrating given that summer is a wonderful time to be a Montrealer. I absolutely loved how this city came to life in the warm weather, and I enjoyed making the most of it.

However, in the summer of 2004, I was in the depths of another debilitating depressive episode, and quickly realized I wasn't able to work through it the way I did in February and March. Leaving the apartment—let alone getting through a full work day—was becoming impossible.

This realization, combined with the psychologist's comments, forced me to recognize that my depression may, in fact, be clinical, and would therefore need medical treatment. There was just no other possible explanation.

Years of self-stigma held me back from considering any medical treatment beyond talk therapy, which had delayed my diagnosis and treatment. Finally, I was able to break free of the stigma. I began to regard my illness as what it was—an *illness*.

I asked myself the questions, "How would I be acting and reacting if my heart defect had come back? Would I suffer in silence for years before seeking treatment? Would I feel guilty, ashamed, or 'less than?' Would I be afraid to discuss what was happening to me with family, friends, or colleagues?"

Of course not.

This realization was a watershed moment for me. To this day, it saddens me that I wasted all that time under the spell of stigma, which was fueled by my ignorance and fear. It also hurts that I had to be in such a desperate state before finally shedding the self-stigma holding me back. I have often wondered if being male contributed to the problem. While I've never been afraid of my emotions in any way, the research does show that men are far less likely to speak openly about mental illness than women.

How did I respond to this realization? One day on my way to work, I got off the bus in front of the Montreal General Hospital. I walked into the emergency room and sat in front of the triage nurse. She asked me what was wrong, and I said, "I think I am suffering from clinical depression. It is very severe."

"Are you suicidal?" she asked.

"No. But I'm unable to function and can't work," I said.

"Wait over there. You will be seen soon," she replied.

Private Consultation

Over the years, I've heard many horror stories about hospital emergency wards being ill-suited to respond to urgent cases of mental illness. Our system doesn't always provide the care it should for those suffering from mental illnesses. For some reason, perhaps luck, my visit to the hospital that day went smoothly. Within forty-five minutes of checking in, I was in a private consultation with a psychiatrist. Kind and thorough, she interviewed me for well over an hour.

> **Author's Note:** I am keenly aware of how fortunate I was, and that for many, this option has presented problems. However, if you are in urgent need of care due to severe symptoms of mental illness—and particularly if you're experiencing suicidal thoughts—make a call to a help line or go in person to the emergency room of your local hospital. Even if you face a long wait, saving your life is worth it!

After hearing my story to that point, she explained that although it was too early to diagnose me as having bipolar disorder, she confirmed I was indeed suffering a severe depressive episode. I would need both treatment and a leave of absence from work. She wrote a note indicating three months of sick leave effective immediately and prescribed an antidepressant called Effexor. Then she referred me to the Allen Institute of Montreal, where a psychiatrist would follow my case.

Feeling numb and shocked, I went home and slept the rest of the day. I had just entered a frightening new phase of my life—one that included a diagnosis of mental illness.

After several weeks, the medication took effect and my severe depression abruptly stopped. My first instinct was to be hopeful and optimistic, and I believed I had found a treatment that worked for me. Since this was my first time ever on a leave of absence from work, I was eager to return as soon as possible after my depression subsided. However, my doctor insisted I wait several more weeks before agreeing I was ready.

An Awkward and Terrifying Return

Returning to work was both awkward and terrifying because of the pervasive stigma surrounding my illness. In that moment, I had to focus on how good it felt to be well enough to return to work. I hoped the worst of this experience was behind me. Although I had taken a long time to admit I had a mental illness and consider treatment, I was facing my situation and responding well to the medication. Happily, I experienced a stronger sense of hope than I had felt in years.

Unfortunately, that optimism was premature. In fact, the worst was yet to come.

After only a few weeks back at work, I woke up to the deepest, darkest, and most severe depression I had experienced so far. Without question, I felt more ill than ever. With bone-crushing fatigue affecting me on a cellular level, I was like a zombie. It seemed my brain was under the effect of a powerful sedative, and finding words to describe how I felt was impossible. In fact, were I to attempt writing this paragraph while in that state, it would have taken days—if it could have happened at all.

This was also the most emotionally sad I had felt during a depressive phase. In addition to all of the numbness and distancing and sense of being "shut off," I was acutely aware that I had lost all the optimism I'd experienced the previous weeks. I would need to go on another sick leave, which was devastating to me.

This was the first time I honestly asked the questions, "Will I ever feel normal? Will I feel like *me* again?" Instead of thinking I was turning a corner and getting some measure of control over my illness, I faced the toughest challenge of my life, and I had no clear sense of the outcome. It was terrifying.

After telling my manager I was experiencing a relapse, I consulted my psychiatrist. He increased the dosage of Effexor based on these key facts: I was clearly in another severe depressive episode; the Effexor had shown signs of effectiveness; and I was still on a moderate dosage with room to increase it safely. Given the circumstances, his decision was reasonable.

Unfortunately for me, Effexor had another, unintended effect. It opened the door to an entirely new aspect of my illness, which would force me to face the greatest obstacle of my life.

THE WORLD OF HYPOMANIA

I've described the depressive episodes I experienced periodically from January 2002 to late 2004. However, that wasn't the entire story. After each episode of clinical depression, my mood would suddenly shift to long periods of hypomania, during which I'd experience the opposite of depression.

In the same way that clinical depression has a spectrum from mild to moderate to severe, mania also has a spectrum. Mild and moderate mania is called hypomania, while severe mania is called mania, or a manic episode. According to NAMI (National Alliance on Mental Illness): "Hypomania is a milder form of mania that doesn't include psychotic episodes. People with hypomania can often function well in social situations or at work. Some people with bipolar disorder will have episodes of mania or hypomania many times throughout their life; others may experience them only rarely."

Hypomania Came on Suddenly

My first hypomanic episode, which was mild, came in March 2002 after my first depressive episode abruptly ended. These transitions—from feeling well in 2001 to depressed and then mildly hypomanic in early 2002—came on suddenly as I slept. I would go to bed feeling one way and wake up feeling entirely different. It was disorienting, to say the least.

At the time, I had absolutely no idea I was hypomanic; in fact, I didn't know what that word meant. All I knew was the symptoms of depression (or that mystery flu, as I thought at the time) were gone and I felt good again. Mild hypomania is actually quite close to a stable mood, with only subtle and hard-to-diagnose symptoms. For example, I needed one to two fewer hours of sleep each night, but this change was easy to dismiss. I had more energy than normal, but nothing excessive. I just felt "on" in every way. After being depressed for two months, I must admit, this hypomanic phase felt fantastic!

In hindsight, the problem with my state was one of sustainability. It's not possible for anyone to sustain hypomania and be healthy. We're not meant to suddenly need fewer hours of sleep at night or have a markedly higher output of productivity and energy every day, all day. We need to rest and recoup. But I didn't do that, because my energy was constant. Even my sleep felt strangely energetic.

Another problem with hypomania involves decision making, which can become impulsive. The first evidence of bipolar disorder symptoms was an incident that had clearly affected my behavior. This incident happened a few years before the onset of continuous symptoms, and it involved one uncharacteristic decision I made when I was twenty-four. I traded in the car I owned for a new lease, which admittedly doesn't seem strange. But for me, it was.

Up to that point, I had established a clear pattern of behavior when it came to large financial decisions—that is, I'd seek my dad's advice. We had always been close, and his advice helped me tremendously. I was grateful to have a father in my life who enjoyed helping me this way, so asking him made sense. However, on this occasion, I suddenly had the idea I wanted a new car, despite the fact I couldn't afford the payments. Within a few days, I had selected the car I wanted and accepted a trade-in on my existing one. I signed the paperwork, picked up my new car, and only then called Dad.

It turned out I had overpaid for this new car and was severely underpaid for the trade-in on my old car. Dad was quite surprised I had made these decisions without chatting with him first—not for his approval, but for his helpful guidance. He could have stopped me from making this mistake, and in doing so, saved me a significant amount of money.

This was the first time hypomania had directly affected my behavior—and thus my life.

Is Hypomania Fun?

When I deliver my keynote lectures, I'm often asked if my hypomania was fun. It's a fair question. Although having excess energy is, in principle, a great deal better than having low or zero energy, hypomania is not fun at all. Despite the seductive and seemingly endless energy, we all need rest on a cellular level, and hypomania won't let us get it. To live on an unsustainable high is both exhausting and disorienting.

With hypomania, you know (even subconsciously) you are racing towards a cliff. For me, that cliff came in the form of my next depressive episode.

Defining Moderate Hypomania

As with my successive depressive episodes that continually became more severe, my recurring hypomanic episodes gradually moved from mild to moderate. Earlier, I described mild hypomania as something relatively difficult to diagnose or even notice if you don't know what to look for. Moderate hypomania, however, is an entirely different thing.

My moderate hypomania was immediately apparent to everyone in my life. My girlfriend, my friends, my colleagues, and my boss all noticed I was operating on some sort of "high." I suddenly found myself with access to an endless torrent of pure energy. As a result, my need for sleep dropped all the way down to four or five hours a night—the least I had ever required.

Another dramatic change in my behavior came in the form of my early morning jogging on Mount Royal Park. On its own, the thought of a young man jogging every morning before work isn't all that remarkable. However, I absolutely hated running and had never jogged a day in my life! I started doing it because I needed a way to clear my mind and burn some of this energy I suddenly had on tap. So after only four or five hours of sleep, I would run for one or two hours in the early morning before work.

Remember, this was happening in April 2004 to a man who, only weeks before, had been in the throes of a severe depression. The contrast was jarring, and the impact of my moderate hypomania spilled into my work performance as well.

In truth, mild hypomania wasn't quite noticeable at work because the outward signs were so close to my baseline personality. The only real indicators were the twenty-four-hour sustainability of my energy and the sudden change in my sleep and rest patterns, which my colleagues and managers couldn't see.

Moderate hypomania, however, was much more obvious. Suddenly I was too eager, too hyper, too talkative, too willing to take on extra projects, and my focus and ability to complete projects with any attention to detail were clearly impaired. My manager asked me several times over a few months to stay focused and finish the task at hand rather than work on another project. This had never happened before; I had long established an excellent track record of finishing projects well, with keen attention to detail.

Only one person in my life, my fiancée at the time, had any clue a pattern in my symptoms was emerging. And that pattern indicated the potential for bipolar disorder, which meant I was at risk for a manic episode.

That is exactly what happened in February 2005.

A TSUNAMI OF ENERGY

Earlier, I described how an extremely severe depressive episode resulted in my psychiatrist increasing the dosage of Effexor. I would later learn that, in some cases of patients with bipolar disorder, certain antidepressants, including Effexor, could initiate a manic episode. This proved true for me.

In January 2005, I was not yet diagnosed with bipolar disorder, as I had never experienced a manic episode, and I was in a depressive state so severe that the doctor was forced to treat the symptoms that were presenting. This was more a matter of bad luck than bad management.

Nonetheless, I took the prescribed increase of Effexor the same day I saw my psychiatrist. I was two weeks into the most recent—and most severe—depressive episode and was already reaching the limits of what I could bear. I hoped the increase would give me some relief. After taking it, I went to bed.

I woke up at 1:30 that morning, riding a tsunami of energy unlike anything I had ever felt. Electricity was racing through my body and mind, and I had a sense that anything and everything was possible.

Although I had been moderately hypomanic before, this was something completely different. One way to put how I felt in perspective is this: As I shared earlier in this book, I had been an avid skydiver. I had completed 168 jumps, including a high-altitude jump from twenty-two thousand feet and a night skydive. As you can imagine, an adrenaline rush comes with such activities. And I was familiar with how that felt.

On this early morning in late January 2005, the sensation coursing through my body made the adrenaline rush after skydiving seem like a post-coffee buzz. I was simultaneously aware that I wasn't well, that I wasn't thinking straight—and that I was capable of almost anything. I felt more creative than ever and had a sense of urgency that I needed to be doing something. I wasn't sure what yet, but after weeks of prison-like depression, I felt an overwhelming desire to run like the wind.

So while my fiancée slept, I made the snap decision to go see my family. That alone doesn't seem all that odd; however, my family lived in Orillia and Penetanguishene, Ontario—a full seven-hour drive from our apartment in Montreal. (Penetanguishene, also known as Penetang, is two hours north of Toronto on the shores of Georgian Bay, which is part of Lake Huron.) You can imagine the confusion and disorientation when she woke to see me frantically packing a bag. Just a few hours before, I'd been at the lowest depths of the worst depression I'd ever experienced. Here I was, giddily telling her I wanted to visit my family.

"Now?" she replied, incredulously.

"Yeah, why not? I feel great!" I responded with way too much energy and enthusiasm.

She tried to stop me, but I refused to change my mind and ultimately left Montreal early that cold winter morning to drive to Orillia. That was the start of a six-day manic episode during which I literally did not stop, not even to rest or sleep. Six days of zero sleep would have a dramatically negative impact on a completely healthy person. In my case, it exacerbated my overall state.

Odd, Intense Behavior

As you might imagine, a manic episode is a strange and frightening thing to experience. Your attention span shortens, you get easily irritated, and you become a terrible, one-sided conversationalist. Ultimately, mania can ruin relationships due to the odd, intense behavior that suddenly appears.

For many people, a manic episode can have catastrophic results because of the erosion of awareness and decision-making ability. Some spend or gamble away enormous sums, often money leveraged from credit. Others try to slow their manic episode with alcohol or drugs, often in volumes and types they would never take normally. Some cheat on their spouses or engage in high-risk sexual activity with strangers or prostitutes. Others engage in street or bar fights when normally they would never do such a thing.

These things happen because, during a manic episode, two very dangerous ingredients mix: a massive excess of physical and mental energy along with a quickly eroding sense of reality.

Still, 144 hours of being awake over six days was a very long time to fill. While I managed to avoid the more destructive aspects of mania, I was not immune to its strange parts.

> **Author's Note:** As I look back on my manic episode, I realize how incredibly lucky I was. My research regarding bipolar disorder indicates that manic episodes often include the extreme or damaging behavior described above. Thankfully, my behavior never fell into those traps. I can't claim I had any control over avoiding the worst behaviors, because I didn't feel I had much control at all; I chalk it up to plain old luck. Maybe this was a bit of the luck my father (and Stephen Leacock) said I'd have if I worked hard and lived life with tenacity and persistence. I'll always be grateful that this manic episode wasn't more destructive.

Surprised My Oldest Brother

One of my many strange behaviors happened upon my arrival in Orillia that first morning.

During the long drive from Montreal, I had come up with the idea to surprise my oldest brother by showing up at his workplace. And that's exactly what I did. When he arrived that morning, his little brother from Montreal was waiting in the parking lot in front of his office. Understandably surprised and confused, he asked if anything was wrong, to which I said, "No, but I would love to go for a drive with you. Can you take some time off work?"

He kindly agreed, and we drove around for several hours, during which he was barely able to get a word in edgewise. Although I'd always been accurately described as "chatty," it was unusual for me to dominate a conversation in this way. He could tell something was wrong with me, but understandably had no idea what was happening. As my oldest brother, he always looked out for me when he could, but this may have been the hardest I'd leaned on him. Although he was confused and certainly worried, he handled the situation with patience and care for me.

The next several days of my manic episode are somewhat blurred, with only certain moments clear in my memory. All of them amount to highly strange behavior, and I can only imagine the confusion, uncertainty, and ultimately concern it caused my family.

Here are a few specific incidents I remember clearly.

Hot Tub Yoga

During the first few days of my manic episode, I stayed with my oldest brother and my sister-in-law, who have a hot tub on their deck. At one point, I went out to the hot tub to try to relax. However, after just a few minutes alone in the tub, I became distracted and bored. So I got out and began doing yoga-style poses and exercises on the deck. This was especially unusual given that it was the middle of a typical Canadian winter, and the temperature was minus twenty degrees Celsius.

My sister-in-law saw this out of her kitchen window and, after briefly watching me in total confusion, she had to ask me to get back in the tub. I didn't even notice I was cold.

While this was a relatively harmless moment during my manic episode, I often think of how disorienting it must have been for her to find me behaving in such a strange way—especially because at the time none of us knew about my illness.

Starry Snow Angels

When I wasn't staying with my brother and sister-in-law in Orillia, I was with my dad and his girlfriend in Penetanguishene. One night, Dad stayed up late with me, patiently answering random questions and just letting me talk. He asked me to try to sleep, as he knew it had been days at this point, and I agreed I would try. But I just couldn't; the energy running through my body and mind was like an electrical current that had been turned on and wouldn't turn off.

Their home was across from Penetanguishene Bay, which at that time of year was frozen over. I quietly got up, dressed for the cold, and walked across the street and onto the ice. I followed a snowmobile track for long time, probably walking a mile or more, and then I stepped twenty feet or so off the trail and onto the untouched snow. It was a beautifully clear night, and the stars were brilliant. I lay down on my back in the snow and made a snow angel while looking up at the night sky and weeping at its beauty. Every once in a while, I got up and moved a few feet so I could make a fresh snow angel. I must have made twenty of them before I finally walked back. I have often thought about how puzzling it must have been for the snowmobiler or ice fisherman who found those snow angels the next day!

The Tim Horton's Genius

The nights were the hardest; there was so much time to fill while everyone else was asleep. One of my favorite things to do—which helped me get through several manic nights—was to sit in a corner of one of the local Tim Horton's, a ubiquitous coffee and donut shop in the area, and let my creativity flow. I would order a coffee, which in hindsight could not have been a worse beverage choice, and ask for a stack of Tim Horton's paper placemats, which were blank on one side.

After ignoring the confused look of the staff, I would sit and write out the many ideas racing through my mind. A common part of a manic episode is heightened creativity combined with a growing delusion of grandeur. I had ideas for screenplays that Hollywood would absolutely buy and produce. I had ideas for businesses that would make me a millionaire before age thirty, which I would turn on July 31st of that year. I wrote poetry. I wrote ideas for novels. I wrote until I had pages and pages of notes, which I kept protectively.

However, by this point in my manic episode, I was losing my connection with reality. This was proven weeks later when I looked at my illegible notes—the output of my genius—and realized they read like a puzzle of incomplete thoughts and unrealistic ideas.

The following images are scans of two of my pages of notes. The first shows my brainstorming for a screenplay I was convinced I would not only write, but that would bring me fame and fortune in Hollywood. The second shows my anger, denial, and misguided plans to sue Soldiers' Memorial Hospital (where I was initially admitted) for malpractice. More on that shortly.

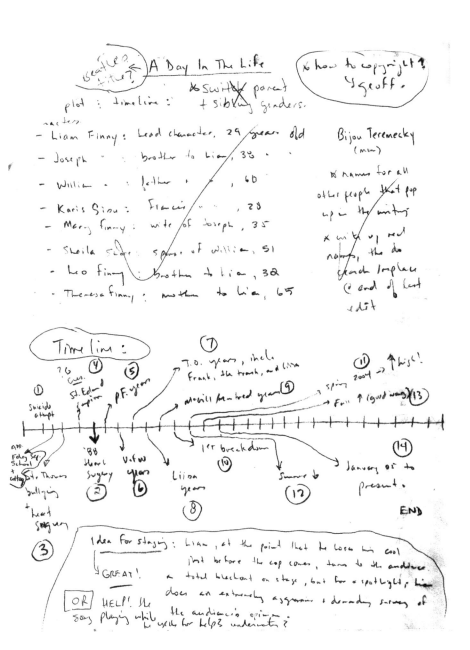

Beatles title? → A Day In The Life   ✗ how to copyright? ✓ geoff.

plot : timeline :   ✗ Switch parent + sibling genders.

characters
- Liam Finny : Lead character, 29 years old   Bijou Teremecky (mm)
- Joseph   "   : brother to Liam, 33 .
- William "   : father to   "   , 60   ✗ names for all other people that pop up in the writing
- Karis Siou : Frances "   " , 28   ✗ with vj real names, the do
- Mary Finny : wife of Joseph , 35   a search implace
- Sheila Siou : spouse of William, 51   @ end of last edit
- Leo Finny : brother to Liam, 32
- Theresa Finny : mother to Liam, 65

Timeline :

① Suicide attempt
② '88 Heart Surgery
③ ABD Foley Sec School + cottage St. Thomas bullying + heart surgery
④ 76 cur. St. Edward baptism
⑤ P.F. years
⑥ U.F.W years
⑦ T.O. years, incl. Frank, the trash, and Lisa
⑧ Lisa years
⑨ Montreal Montreal years
⑩ 1st breakdown
⑪ 2004 → this!
⑫ Summer 6
⑬ Fall ↑ (gud was)
⑭ January 05 to present.

END

Idea for staging: Liam, at the point that he loses his cool just before the cop comes, turns to the audience. a total blackout on stage, but for a spotlight, Liam does an extremely aggressive + demanding survey of the audience's opinion.

↳ GREAT!

OR HELP! He song playing while he yells for help? undersets? the

· MALPRACTICE SUIT — SOLDIER'S

Firm: Ralston
Lawyer: Keating
Referred: Ray J.
Morton

MAIN FAILURES OF JUDGEMENT :

① to commit me involuntarily via a Form 1 when I was clearly able to speak in a calm, logical manner — so long as I was given the opportunity to do so for more than 10 sec. ☆

② The decision to override the prescription of my 187.5mg   MH Dr. Blean
of Effexox each day and make me cease taking the medication "cold turkey". No "weaning period" was even mentioned

☆ Facts : while I was visibly agitated, raising my voice, speaking quickly and interrupting frequently (often demanding a "yes" or "no" answer), I was NOT being physically aggressive/threatening to anyone, including myself. I believe this to be the core of my case: I was agitated, yes, but was begging, with a soft, tremulous voice, to be heard, and NO ONE (family or medical staff) would even entertain the idea of hearing my side of the story (let alone considering the validity of my claims

The Hospital Near Miss

As my manic episode progressed, it was clear to everyone in my family that I was not well. But no one, me included, had any idea of exactly what was happening. My fiancée, stuck back in Montreal and trying to manage the situation from there, was the only one who understood that I was, in fact, suffering a manic episode. She was in regular contact with me and my family, trying to get all of us to understand the seriousness of the situation.

I was able to grasp the reality that something was wrong and even correctly guessed the Effexor had initiated this manic phase. For this reason, I had stopped taking Effexor on the second day, and then on the fourth night, I sought medical help. I went to the Orillia Soldiers' Memorial Hospital emergency room late one night and asked to see a psychiatrist. I believed that only a psychiatrist would be able to help me.

Unfortunately, there wasn't a psychiatrist on staff that night, but I was told one was on duty at the Royal Victoria Hospital in Barrie, a half hour's drive south of Orillia. Because I had decided to seek help, I made the drive to Barrie and informed the triage nurse at Royal Victoria that I wished to see a psychiatrist. After completing the triage process, I was asked to wait. However, in my state, patience was on short supply, so over the course of an hour, I asked several times for a progress update. I'm sure the triage nurse found me frustrating. Finally, she snapped at me, saying quite firmly, "Just be patient and wait your turn! I will call you when the doctor is available!"

Fully manic at this point, I was unable to process my reaction, just as I couldn't summon the patience to wait for the doctor. Despite it being the worst thing for my own well-being, I was overwhelmed with anger. Indignantly, I stormed out of the hospital. I finished that night at a nearby Tim Horton's, adding to my stack of brilliant notes.

Mad at Dad

Let me begin by saying that my dad and I are extremely close and always have been. We are as much friends as we are father and son. He has always been there for me, and I've had very few reasons to be upset at him in my entire life.

However, for reasons I will never understand, nearly all the anger that spilled out of me during my manic episode was directed at my dad. I remember twice being on the phone with him and something he said set me off. In both cases, I screamed at him. Full-on rage screams, swearing a blue streak, not letting him get in a word. It amazes me to this day that he had the presence of mind to know this wasn't me, and he didn't engage at all. He didn't defend himself or lash back; he only tried to calm me down and keep me talking as he worked towards understanding what on earth was happening to his son.

There are many things I did during my manic episode that are embarrassing, and some I wish I could take back, but none that make me feel the shame and regret I feel for what I put my father through in those moments. I am forever grateful he was able to instantly forgive me for my actions. He understood they were beyond my control. His lack of stigma, his poise, patience, empathy, and love in those terrible moments have been among the greatest gifts of my life.

THE INTERVENTION

Over the course of the final night and day of my manic episode, it was becoming clear to everyone that my mental state was unravelling, and I needed help. The fact that I'd attempted to admit myself to the hospital showed I was somewhat aware, but leaving the hospital showed I didn't possess the patience needed to do it on my own. So my family, with consistent input from my fiancée in Montreal, arranged an intervention to get me into the hospital—against my will, if necessary.

It would take me months to fully grasp the enormity of their action, and to this day, I can't entirely imagine how hard it must have been. But there was no denying it was needed, as I indeed fit the description of potentially "posing harm to myself or others," which is the legal requirement to admit a person against their will.

While I was not suicidal and had not exhibited direct violence towards others, the fact that I had not slept in five days and was driving my car during the day and night was a major concern. If I were allowed to go on for much longer, the chances of having an accident or losing control of my anger and becoming violent would increase.

The plan was simple. My dad invited me to lunch with my high school sweetheart's parents, who were still dear friends all these years later, and arranged for the local police to arrive at a set time. By then, my behavior had devolved to the point where it was extremely uncomfortable to be around me. I did not let anyone at that table speak at all. I wanted to express how I was thinking and feeling, and I wanted to do it my way. I said, "If you can sit quietly for two hours watching a movie, why can't you sit quietly and listen to me for five minutes?"

At the time, this made perfect sense to me. I had no idea why they wouldn't just do as I said. But when I look back on this pivotal lunch meeting, I am struck by how awful it must have been for them; here was their son and friend behaving in ways never seen before, and clearly not well. They were all so patient and kind, and they never wavered in their intention to help me.

As we finished eating, my dad said he wanted to go outside for a cigarette and asked me to join him. As I stepped outside, I noticed the police cruiser parked ominously out front, and the officer behind the wheel immediately got out of the car. Strangely, as far removed from normalcy and reality as I was, I instantly knew what was happening. Miraculously, I wasn't upset at all—in fact, I felt relieved. I took a step towards the officer and asked in a friendly voice, "Are you here for Jason Finucan?"

Looking bemused (likely because he expected resistance), the officer replied, "Yes, as a matter of fact, I am. Is that you?"

"Yes, officer, that's me. So front seat or back?" I asked.

Looking even more bemused, he replied, "Well, you should probably get in the back."

I don't remember if I said goodbye to my dad or my friends or if I just left, but after settling into the police car, I asked the officer if it would be okay for me to lie down. "This is my hometown. I went high school here. I would rather not be seen in the back of a police car." He was fine with that, and it's how I spent the only ride I've ever had in the back of a police car—lying down on the back seat on the way to the hospital. Ironically, the nearest hospital was Orillia Soldiers' Memorial where I had previously tried to admit myself but was told there wasn't a psychiatrist on staff that night.

Once we arrived at the hospital, the officer escorted me past the emergency triage to a pre-arranged room in the emergency ward. My family was all there, offering me support and ensuring this process went smoothly. I recall trying to convince the emergency doctor I didn't need to be admitted; I only needed rest. I was selling him hard on the idea that I would check myself into a hotel and sleep—that was all I needed at this point. Thankfully, he wasn't buying, and along with my family, he signed the legal document that, in Ontario at the time, was required to admit adults to a hospital against their will. It resulted in a mandatory minimum two-week stay in a psychiatric hospital from which I could not leave.

The fact that this step was necessary—and the best thing for me—didn't make what came next any easier.

The following is a scan of the form used to admit me that day.

Ministry of Health | Form 42 *Mental Health Act* | Notice to Person under Subsection 38.1 of the Act of Application for Psychiatric Assessment under Section 15 or an Order under Section 32 of the Act

Ontario

Part I *(complete only if appropriate)*

To: _Jason William Finucan_
(name of person)

of _4105 Cote des Neiges Montreal_
(home address)

This is to inform you that _Dr. T.R. Lobsinger._
(name of physician)

examined you on _8 Feb 2005_
(date of examination) (day / month / year)

and has made an application for you to have a psychiatric assessment.

Part A and/or Part B must be completed

Part A

That physician has certified that he/she has reasonable cause to believe that you have:

Check Box(es)

☐ threatened or attempted or are threatening or attempting to cause bodily harm to yourself;

☐ behaved or are behaving violently towards another person or have caused or are causing another person to fear bodily harm from you; or

☒ shown or are showing a lack of competence to care for yourself.

and that you are suffering from a mental disorder of a nature or quality that likely will result in:

Check Box(es)

☐ serious bodily harm to yourself;

☐ serious bodily harm to another person; or

☒ serious physical impairment of you.

Part B

That physician has certified that he/she has reasonable cause to believe that you:

a) have previously received treatment for mental disorder of an ongoing or recurring nature that, when not treated, is of a nature or quality that likely will result in

☐ serious bodily harm to yourself,

☐ serious bodily harm to another person,

☐ substantial mental or physical deterioration of you, or

☐ serious physical impairment of you;

b) have shown clinical improvement as a result of the treatment;

c) are suffering from the same mental disorder as the one for which you previously received treatment or from a mental disorder that is similar to the previous one;

(Disponible en version française)   *See reverse*

787–41 (00/12)*   7530–4627

The Psych Ward—Part 1

The psych ward is a term I'd heard many times in my life, mostly related to movies such as *One Flew Over the Cuckoo's Nest*. Occasionally, it referred to distant family members or friends of a friend who had "lost their mind" and spent time in the "psych ward." At any rate, as far as I was concerned, being in one wasn't good.

After my family members signed the forms and my admission was complete, they had nothing to do but leave and hope. I had been put in the care of the psychiatric ward of the hospital, which in Soldiers' Memorial amounted to one highly unique room. The reality of my situation began to sink in when I was escorted into that room and noticed several odd things. For one, I saw an armed security guard seated in a chair just outside the door.

At first, I wondered who this guard was protecting me from, since no one knew I was there except my family. It was jarring to realize her job was to protect everyone outside the room from *me*. Inside the room, which smelled of leather and bleach, were padded walls, a sparse bathroom with no door and no sharp edges anywhere, and a pedestal bed with leather straps on each side.

I was informed I would spend the night here and then transfer the next day to the Penetanguishene Mental Health Centre (now Waypoint Mental Health Centre). People often referred to this hospital as "the nut house," and its location became a common joke in the area. For example, they'd say things like "he's losing his marbles; if he doesn't come around, he'll be sent to Penetang." Suddenly, these seemingly innocuous jokes held a very different meaning.

The nurse in charge of me at Soldiers' suggested I take a sedative to help me rest, which was absolutely needed. Unfortunately, one of the few things I knew for certain was that a drug, Effexor, had put me in this state, so my instinct was to reject any more medication. I made my case to the nurse very emphatically and apparently convincingly, because she made me a deal.

"I will agree not to give you a shot, but you have to lie down and rest. Okay?"

"Okay, I will," I replied.

And I did for as long as I could, which was somewhere between twenty minutes and an hour. Then I sat up and started chatting with the security guard. At first, she was on edge while ascertaining if I was a flight risk. But then she relaxed when it was clear I just wanted to talk. She was very kind, and at one point she said I should try to sleep.

The next thing I knew, I was waking up and it was dark. I don't know how much time had passed, but likely a few hours. I do know it was the first sleep of any kind I'd had in six days. What I didn't know was where I was. I genuinely had no clue. The room looked strange to me, like I'd never seen it before. I got up and walked to the window to get an idea of my location. I saw a house my oldest brother used to rent across the street, which confused me even more. Through my brain fog, I wondered, "Why am I seeing my brother's house? Why from this angle? Where am I?"

As these thoughts floated through my foggy mind, I was suddenly startled by a terse voice.

"Go back to bed, Mr. Finucan."

I turned away from the window and, to my shock, saw multiple people gathered near the doorway. There were four nurses, four male orderlies, and the security guard. They all looked upset—at the very least extremely tense.

"What's wrong? Did I do something wrong?" I asked, totally confused.

"Just go BACK to bed, Mr. Finucan. NOW," someone replied, sounding more agitated.

"Okay, but will someone please tell me what's happening?" I asked as I walked back to the bed and sat down.

The second I sat down, the four male orderlies and some of the nurses pounced on me. I was forcibly held down by certain hands while others quickly connected the leather straps until I was tightly bound to the bed. During this process, I got extremely upset and remember yelling things like "Why are you doing this to me?" and "I didn't do anything wrong! What did I do to deserve this?"

In the midst of all of this, I noticed the face of one of the orderlies. What caught my attention was that he didn't look stern or upset. Instead, his face was filled with empathy and sadness. And then I realized why.

I knew him, and he knew me.

He was the father of a girl I went to high school with, and was close friends with my high school sweetheart's parents. It was especially painful to recognize someone I knew when I was in such a vulnerable place. And it was confusing to feel unjustly violated in this way, to be strapped to a bed when, as far as I understood, I had done nothing to warrant it. The fact that he looked so concerned for me—he clearly did not like doing this—was both comforting and confusing.

As soon as I was strapped down, the nurse who had made the deal with me said, "I agreed to no medication if you would stay in bed and rest; since you can't, I have to give you this to help you sleep." A needle was plunged into my thigh, and I fell almost immediately into a deep sleep.

The Psych Ward—Part 2

The next morning, still feeling extremely groggy from the sedative, I was transferred by ambulance to the Penetanguishene Mental Health Centre. "Nut house," my subconscious reminded me. "You're being sent to Penetang," it continued.

> **Author's Note:** Although my knowledge of the Penetanguishene Mental Health Centre at the time was highly negative and stigmatized, it is in fact a top-tier hospital that provides excellent care to people suffering from acute and severe mental illnesses. My thoughts at the time were left over from years of stigma towards mental illness.

My mood briefly lifted when the paramedic riding with me in the back of the ambulance asked if I liked the movie *The Pirates of the Caribbean*. "Sure," I replied, "but why do you ask?"

"I can play it for you, to pass the time. We won't be in Penetang for forty-five minutes," he explained.

Only then did I notice the small LCD TV mounted near the back doors of the ambulance. Childlike, I spent the remainder of the drive watching Captain Jack Sparrow do his thing, bemused that I was watching a movie in the back of an ambulance. For a few minutes, I actually forgot where I was going.

Once we arrived, reality came crashing in. The nurses who greeted me explained that because I was being transferred on a forced admission, I would need to be placed in the lockdown ward until the resident psychiatrist could consult with me. The problem was, it was a Friday and he had already left for the weekend, so the earliest I could see him was

Monday. That meant I had to spend the next two days and three nights in a lockdown ward reserved for the most ill and the most aggressive patients in the hospital.

At approximately two thousand square feet, this sparse-looking ward was divided into two sleeping rooms. The twin beds were arranged in rows with nothing between them, like a barracks, and there were a few other rooms for living space. I saw some books and games, but not much else. The patients in there with me were extremely ill, suffering from severe mental illnesses. Their behavior ranged from bizarre to highly aggressive, and while no one was directly abusive to me, I felt incredibly uncomfortable the whole time. Although no one's actions made me feel unsafe, it was difficult to not be afraid, given the movie reel of images running through my mind of people in psych wards being violent.

For example, the man in the bed beside mine had terrible night terrors. He'd wake up a few times at night, sit up, and scream as though he were being torn apart. It was the most painful, guttural scream I had ever heard. Thankfully, he went back to sleep fairly quickly, but as you can imagine, it was hard for me to get any rest.

There was also a young woman who had a delusion that we were in a communist prison held unjustly against our will. She had come up with a plan for us to break free. Each day for the three days I was in that lockdown ward, she'd explain all of this to me, including how we had to tackle the nurse when she brought our dinner so we could make a run for it. Given her intensity in sharing these plans with me, I was amazed she never acted.

One other fellow patient was a young man, perhaps twenty years old, who seemed to be suffering from narcissistic delusions of grandeur. He spoke constantly about how he had god-like powers and could control the outside world with his thoughts. Charming and extremely intense, he appeared to believe every word he said.

The following image is a scan of one of the drawings he handed me one day, unprompted. I don't share this information or the image to be insensitive to his condition, but rather to provide color and detail on the experience I faced at that time.

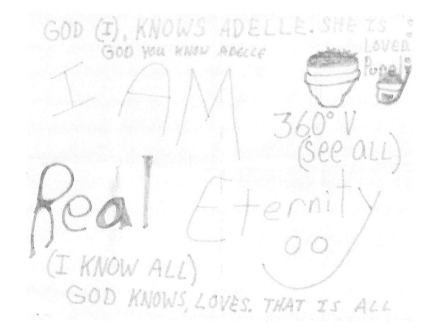

Mostly, I kept to myself and tried to come to terms with the reality that, on some level, I belonged there. That thought terrified me, though, because it seemed clear that most of my seriously ill fellow patients were unlikely to recover. What hope did I have? Although I wondered this, I didn't despair; I just tried to focus on my Monday meeting with the doctor that couldn't come soon enough.

Here's another factor that made these days the longest of my life: Zyprexa. That was the anti-psychotic drug I was given to help me come down from the manic episode. Although effective in treating mania, Zyprexa has side effects that are nothing short of terrible. I experienced constant hunger, even immediately after eating a full meal, that led to overeating and rapid weight gain. In the two months I was on it, I went from 190 pounds to 215 pounds.

While on that medication, I had a constant foggy-brained sensation, as if I were just waking up and couldn't quite clear the cobwebs. To top it off, Zyprexa also dulled my sex drive and made me impotent. (This last side effect wasn't evident during my time in hospital, but was an unpleasant surprise when I was back in Montreal and reunited with my fiancée.)

On Monday, I finally found myself sitting in a room with a kind psychiatrist. I don't recall his name, but I do recall he was from India and was exceptionally good at his job. He patiently walked me through a detailed, thorough interview. After collecting the facts of my story and symptoms of my illness to date, he offered a clear diagnosis, Bipolar 1, and a treatment plan, lithium. He viewed taking Effexor as an unfortunate error and said Zyprexa could be dropped in two months.

In every way, I hit my absolute lowest point during this time spent in two different psych wards. I had never been so ill nor so vulnerable, and I had never felt so alone. Whatever support existed for me outside of those walls seemed irrelevant during that long and terrible weekend. I was utterly alone while strapped to that bed, and somehow even more so in that lockdown ward surrounded by other patients. I tried not to think about the possibility that this could become my life; that was too much to bear.

But like the old cliché says, when you hit rock bottom, you have nowhere to go but up. In these two psych wards, I hit my rock bottom, but finally being diagnosed and given a clear course of treatment became the first two rungs in the long ladder I'd climb back to health.

THE SHEER POWER OF STIGMA

My first encounter with stigma came in the form of self-stigma. As it turned out, my attitude had been part of the problem all along. I was among those who considered mental illnesses such as depression as a lack of motivation or a character flaw I didn't respect—and certainly couldn't relate to.

Despite being widely known as an empathetic, caring, and an all-around nice guy, I had spent years quietly judging those in my life who were suffering from mental illness—including my mom, who had suffered from clinical depression for years. To me, these people were lacking in strength, willpower, motivation, and drive. This couldn't happen to me.

My self-stigma was so strong that for nearly two full years, I refused treatment and turned to pure willpower to get myself back to health. As I have described, those two years were marked by extreme swings in my mood from severe depression to mania and everything in between.

The fact that I took so long to face the reality of my illness speaks to the sheer power of stigma. I can imagine a long list of minor illnesses, such as chronic migraines or nausea, that I would have refused to put up with. I certainly wouldn't have tried to live through them, using only willpower and hoping they would improve. Instead, I would have sought treatment and done what was necessary to recover.

Faced with Discrimination

During this time, I was also forced to deal with stigma in a second, external way—in the form of discomfort and at times outright discrimination from those around me. The most common example I heard was, *"Jason, can't you just try harder and snap out of it?"*

Unfortunately, most people in my professional and social life were also struggling with stigma. If my heart defect had resurfaced instead, what was said to me and actions taken towards me would never have happened. Could you imagine saying "just try harder" to a person suffering from a heart defect, breast cancer, or type 1 diabetes? Stigma led to a form of discrimination that caused many people—none of them intending harm—to act strangely towards me.

Now that my brain was failing, all of the support and empathy that came my way when my heart wasn't working was nowhere to be seen. This made no sense to me, but I don't judge or begrudge anyone who fell into the trap of stigma. Until I actually experienced a mental illness, I had made the same mistake—one that I believe societal norms set us up to make.

My ability to understand that fear and a lack of understanding are the root of stigma derives from my combined experiences of a major physical illness and a major mental illness. My heart defect and the utter lack of stigma towards it allowed me to reach a greater level of understanding when faced with the stigma of mental illness.

Although it took two long years of banging my head against a wall, I finally understood that Bipolar 1 was, in fact, an illness, and, in many ways, it was no different than my heart defect. My first step was to respond to it properly—as a medical illness that required my attention, research, and ultimately the right treatment. For me, this approach led to a successful return to health within six months following my brief residence in the two psych wards.

CREATE YOUR
STIGMAZERO WORKPLACE
PART 4

The Paradox Facing Mental Illness Sufferers

People who have well-known physical illnesses enjoy a luxury that doesn't apply to those with a mental illness. If you are diagnosed with heart defect, kidney disease, cancer, diabetes, or any other common illness, most people around you are at least familiar with what's happening to you. That allows for them to feel empathy, and allows you to feel their support. In the majority of cases, they won't judge you for having the illness, and actively stigmatizing your illness likely won't even enter their minds.

When you suffer from a mental illness, however, most people in your life won't understand what you are going through. Whether you have bipolar disorder, as I do, or depression, post-partum depression, anxiety, or any other mental illness, they likely won't have the faintest idea what you're going through. Many will have a kind of stigma in their minds—because of years of misinformation, because of a deep lack of understanding, and because of fear. Some people fear how your illness may change your behavior, while family members may fear the idea that if you have it, they're likely to experience it as well. Others will fear the unknown.

This leads to the most painful paradox facing mental illness sufferers. Across the spectrum of mental illnesses is a wide variety of symptoms; however, one common thread is that our ability to communicate is drastically impaired. It's incredibly hard to explain to others how we're feeling and what our symptoms are truly like.

Do you see the problem?

How can we raise awareness, reduce stigma, and eradicate discrimination among those who struggle to understand a complex mental illness when the most effective way to do so—clear, unemotional, fact-based and accurate communication—challenges those of us who suffer?

As someone diagnosed with a mental illness, I feel compelled to act. I founded StigmaZero to help employers address the complex and challenging reality of workplace mental illness stigma. I share my story through The StigmaZero Online Training Academy, this book and inspirational keynote lectures while also providing my consulting expertise to employers.

My goal has always been the same. *I want to be an active part of the solution to this problem.* I strive to live and see a day when the amount of stigma experienced by someone with a mental illness equals that of a person with cancer: zero.

Awareness Advocates:
Celebrities and the "Rest of Us"

Each January, Bell Canada Enterprises (BCE), Canada's largest telecommunications company, hosts their Let's Talk Day. For years, Bell has been a corporate leader in the effort to raise awareness of mental illness, particularly in the workplace. Its leaders have also placed considerable focus on the need to reduce the stigma that surrounds mental illness. As a mental health advocate and inspirational speaker working to overcome stigma, I applaud the Bell organization for the success of this initiative. It has helped motivate millions to, as their slogan invites, "join the conversation about mental illness."

A key strategy Bell has employed is turning to celebrity advocates for mental health. These brave and inspiring individuals have all experienced mental illness in some way. They are using their platform of fame and Bell's well-known Let's Talk Campaign to create enormous reach. Names like Clara Hughes (Olympic athlete), Michael Landsberg (sports broadcaster), Mary Walsh (comedienne and actress), and Howie Mandel (comedian and TV personality) make up the core of Bell's spokespersons for mental health.

Other well-known celebrities who have joined this movement to end stigma through their own organizations and campaigns are Demi Lovato (American singer, songwriter, and actress), Glenn Close (American actress, singer, and film producer), Dwayne "The Rock" Johnson (American actor and former professional wrestler), and Stephen Fry (British actor, comedian, actor, writer, presenter, and activist), to name a few. Their willingness to speak publicly about their (or their family member's) experiences with mental illness helps many to feel they are not alone. Their outreach also draws attention to the stigma.

Celebrity advocates are only one part of the equation, however. While their willingness to speak out generates respect and admiration, the average person often can't relate to them. Because our society tends to hold celebrities in high regard, we believe their success places them out of our reach. We listen and we admire, but we may not feel empowered to act in our own lives. We perceive we aren't as confident in our abilities when we compare our talents to theirs.

For this reason, I believe all campaigns to raise awareness of mental illness and reduce its stigma must also involve advocates from "the rest of us." We are the non-celebrities who have experienced a mental illness and are willing to speak out about our challenges and our belief that this stigma needs to be eradicated. A combination of celebrity and non-celebrity spokespersons is ideal: a campaign featuring both will have the wide reach of celebrities and the everyman relatability of "the rest of us."

For this reason, everyone who faces the challenge of mental illness needs encouragement to speak out—and to speak out often on any platform they can. The famous can (and should) help to break the ice and draw widespread attention. The rest of us need to take it from there and keep the momentum going.

Most importantly, let's be sure to talk about mental illness not only on Let's Talk Day, but every day.

CHAPTER 3
BECOMING A STIGMA FIGHTER

HITTING ROCK BOTTOM

The first tentative steps of my recovery were taken during my forced stay at the Penetanguishene Mental Health Centre. They began when I was finally given a clinical diagnosis of Bipolar 1 Disorder and a clearly mapped treatment plan. Although I was still very ill and coming down from a manic episode, for the first time in years, I had a clear sense of what illness I was battling. The psychiatrist who provided the diagnosis and prescription of lithium persuaded me that, by being patient and following the treatment plan, I had a good chance of recovery.

Although being formally diagnosed with a major mental illness is terrifying, at that moment I felt relief more than anything. Over several years, I had often used the analogy of "wrestling an octopus in the dark" to describe my experience of living with a mystery illness with no clear diagnosis or treatment plan. Finally having this diagnosis didn't cause me to despair; rather, it gave me hope. This small but powerful kernel of hope fueled me for the next four months. As it turned out, I needed every ounce of that hope as I continued to face huge challenges.

Psych Ward—The Final Chapter
In Chapter 2, I described my experiences in a psychiatric hospital, in particular, the first few days in the lockdown ward. As difficult as those days were, my second week there proved to be the hardest.

By the start of the second week, the Zyprexa I was being given had effectively put out the fire of my manic episode. Although I had returned to a calm state, I still didn't feel at all like myself. Among the many side effects of Zyprexa was a pervasive mental fog, like being awakened from a long nap. I felt slow and confused much of the time. Still, I realized improvement every day.

Interestingly, the more I improved, the harder it was to reconcile my current reality. I was a resident of a mental hospital—against my will.

Even though I started to feel closer to being well enough to leave, I could not be considered for release until the full two weeks were up. The more my recovery progressed, the more trapped I felt. As a result, the last four days felt longer than the first week-and-a-half.

During this time, I did have some visitors; however, the experience was extremely uncomfortable for everyone involved. Mostly, I felt a sense of shame and embarrassment for being there in the first place. The awkward feeling in the room was palpable.

My visitors included my dad and his girlfriend, one of my brothers and my mom, my sister-in-law, my fiancée (who came with her mother), and a friend. They all clearly cared about me and felt empathy for my situation. However, there was an added layer of discomfort, confusion, and of not knowing what to say.

I felt conflicted about having visitors at all. Part of me desperately wanted them to come for the needed support and connection to the real world—one that included a healthy version of me. But another part of me hated seeing them. The looks on their faces only highlighted how bad my situation was.

We were all struggling to manage a situation for which we had active stigma and far too much ignorance. I don't blame anyone for how they acted or didn't act; we were all doing the best we could. But I do believe that if stigma were removed from the equation, the situation would be dramatically improved for everyone.

I believe my experiences with my heart defect and subsequent surgery help to clarify that difference. Then, when friends and family visited me at the hospital, they had empathy and even pity in their eyes, but they still treated me as relatively normal. They understood that something awful and scary was happening to me, something out of my control, and I needed support. I vividly felt all of that love, support, empathy, and most important, lack of discomfort or judgment.

In contrast, when people came to see me at the psychiatric hospital, some of them were clearly uncomfortable and didn't know what to say. Others who would have visited me for a recurrence of my heart problem didn't come at all. Some who did visit looked at me as though I'd changed in a fundamental way. I felt no sense from them that they understood I was sick or facing something out of my control.

As I said earlier, I don't blame anyone for this. We were all in an extreme and difficult situation. Even if you have a clear understanding of mental illness and are free of stigma, seeing a loved one at the tail end of a manic episode is excruciating, because their behavior has been so far out of character. This makes it especially hard to see the illness for what it is rather than judge the person for his or her behavior.

I Saw Myself as Different

Another challenge involved interacting with other patients who were extremely ill and would likely never leave. As I improved, my ability to feel comfortable around them was affected. I couldn't stand their strange behaviors and, in many ways, I needed to see myself as different. I was determined to keep improving; I would recover and definitely leave this hospital. I was not like them.

This thinking wasn't a matter of having a stigma towards them. In fact, I felt enormous empathy for every one of them. However, my survival instincts dictated a need to differentiate myself by seeing a future that included me walking away from that hospital. In many ways, this tenacious frame of mind saved my life.

My Roommate Dave

Another silver lining proved just as important. It came in the form of a new patient named Dave. At the start of my second week, Dave walked through the front door and asked to admit himself. Dave was an alcoholic who had been successfully sober for nearly two years and had recently fallen off the wagon. The combination of this relapse and the guilt and disappointment he felt caused him to become suicidal. The day he admitted himself, he had left his house fully intending to kill himself, but instead chose to seek help.

Unfortunately, there's often a complicated connection between mental illness and addiction to alcohol or drugs. This connection is fueled by stigma.

When people are profoundly suffering from something they can't quite define and, worse, believe they can't talk about openly, they often turn to alcohol or drugs for comfort. That's the trap of "self-medicating"—and it's real and highly dangerous. For some, they'd likely have never had an addiction in the first place were it not for the mental illness. For others, they may have a propensity for an addiction but are in control of it, only to be tripped up by mental illness. In either case, when addiction and mental illness are affecting a person simultaneously, the path to recovery gets much more complex.

Unlike most of the other patients, I was able to connect with Dave. The nurses quickly noticed our similar situations and, on his second night, made us roommates. Dave and I became life preservers for each other, each gaining strength and hope from the other person. We helped each other see that, although we were at a low point, we had every reason to believe in our ability to recover.

During my last few days before being released, Dave and I spent hours walking the grounds—a privilege given to us because we were cleared not to be at risk of fleeing. Although it was winter, it wasn't terribly cold, and the hospital's huge waterfront property was quite beautiful. It had long, plowed walkways from one side of the main building down to the waterfront and back around the other side in a loop. We'd walk a few complete laps of the loop until we got cold and needed to go in.

In our time together, Dave and I shared details about what had led to us being there, and we talked about what we needed to do to recover. For Dave, that meant returning to a regular regimen of AA meetings and therapy sessions—something he'd stopped three months before his relapse because he was doing so well. He was beginning to recognize his addiction to alcohol would require a lifetime of consistent management, and he was making his peace with that.

For me, I knew I had to stay patient as I waited to see if the new lithium treatment would have any positive effect on my illness. I also knew I had to stop feeling stigma towards mental illness, both my own and anyone else's. I resolved to treat my illness with the same diligence and care I'd treat any other major sickness. Like Dave, I had to own it and actively manage it.

OWNING MY ILLNESS

To achieve any meaningful level of recovery, everyone who faces a mental illness must 'own their illness.' Doing so includes overcoming stigma and ultimately passing through the stages of denial and anger to finally reach acceptance. Once all of that dramatic work has been completed, the next phase begins—the one made up of many small but vital tasks. It is during this phase that people begin to fully understand their illness by documenting their symptoms, sleep, and behaviors.

After coming out of a long, intense, and acute phase of bipolar disorder, I was determined to do the work required to fully own my illness. Although I couldn't guarantee I would never suffer a relapse at some point, I knew I could minimize the chances of one by living a balanced lifestyle and doing the tracking work required. I also knew this would better prepare me for a relapse should one occur.

When I started tracking my moods in 2005, I had to retroactively capture the early symptoms I had experienced. Once I caught up, I continued to update my charts and Excel files on a regular basis. Using a resource I found online, I created a simple chart that visually captured my state from severely manic all the way to severely depressed. In addition, I tracked my sleep to ensure I maintained a healthy and steady sleep schedule.

These actions formed the foundation of my expertise on mental illness and stigma. By deciding to actively own and manage my illness—and later to speak openly about my experiences with both physical and mental illnesses—I had taken a huge step forward. Through my work with StigmaZero and this book, I share this expertise with as many people as possible so they can have a better chance to own their illnesses or support those in their life to do the same.

Tracking My Moods and Sleep

The image on the next page comes from the Excel sheet I created. I used this tool to track my mood and sleep using several parameters (hours and quality of sleep, how I felt at wake-up, monthly average weight, sick days, and more). It became an important part of my ability to manage my illness.

2007 Monthly Mood & Sleep Chart for Jason Finucan MAY (190lbs)

Day	1	2	3	4	5	6	7	8	9	10	11	12	13	14	15	16	17	18	19	20	21	22	23	24	25	26	27	28	29	30	31
Hours Slept	6.5	6.5	7.0	7.5	7.0	5.5	5.5	6.5	7.5	8.0	6.5	7.0	7.0	7.0	6.5	7.0	8.5	7.5	6.5	7.0	7.0	5.0	7.0	9.0	8.5	7.0	6.0	6.5	5.5	8.5	7.5
Quality of Sleep - A	1	1	1	1	1	1	1	1	1	1		1	1	1	1	1	1	1	1	1	1	1	1	1	1	1	1	1	1	1	1
Quality of Sleep - B											1																				
Quality of Sleep - C																															
Tired at wake, 100%					1		1							1	1											1		1	1		
less than 100%	1	1	1	1		1		1	1	1	1	1	1			1	1	1	1	1	1	1	1	1	1		1			1	1
Mood - Stable	1	1	1	1	1	1	1	1	1	1	1	1	1	1	1	1	1	1	1	1	1	1	1	1	1	1	1	1	1	1	1
Mood - Depressed 1																															
Mood - Depressed 2																															
Mood - Depressed 3																															
Mood - Manic 1-3																															
Sick day - Bipolar																															
Sick Day - Migraine																															
Sick day - Standard																															
Physical Activity	1	1	1	1	1	1	1	1	1	1	1	1	1	1	1	1	1	1	1	1	1	1	1	1	1	1	1	1	1	1	1

Physical Activity Total:: 31 100%

General Notes:

Daily cough, especially in the morning and at night, lingered for the first two weeks of May, getting (slowly) progressively better until finally disappearing on the 17th.

Totals:

Average h/night Week 1	6.5	
Average h/night Week 2	7.1	
Average h/night Week 3	7.1	
Average h/night Week 4	7.0	
Monthly Average	7.0	
Sick Days - Bipolar	0	#DIV/0!
Sick Days - Migraine	0	#DIV/0!
Sick Days - Standard	0	#DIV/0!
Days of Sleep Quality A	29	94%
Days of Sleep Quality B	2	6%
Days of Sleep Quality C	0	0%
Tired at wake, 100%	8	26%
less than 100%	23	74%
Mood - Stable	31	100%
Mood - Other	0	0%

The following mood and thought charts capture the onset of symptoms of bipolar disorder, including the two years I experienced the most severe symptoms, 2004 and 2005. The baseline indicates my normal level of health, energy, and general function. The shading above or below the baseline shows I was experiencing symptoms related to the states shown on the left.

Mild and moderate mania are also known as "hypomania," while severe mania is known as "manic" or a "manic episode." Depression is generally categorized as mild, moderate, or severe; however, people are likely to experience each of those states differently than I did.

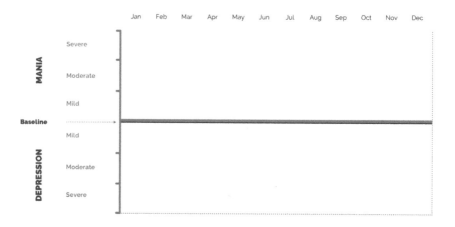

1-Year Life Chart – 2001

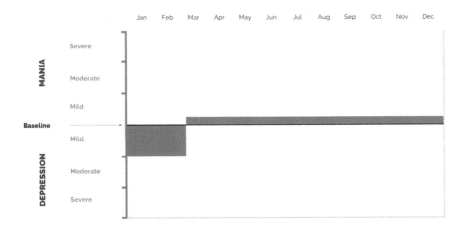

1-Year Life Chart – 2002

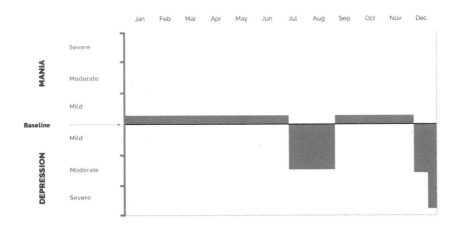

1-Year Life Chart – 2003

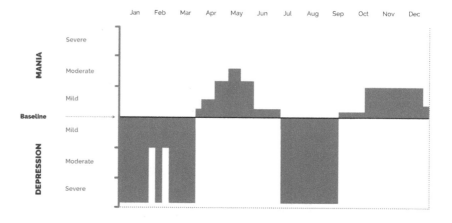

1-Year Life Chart – 2004

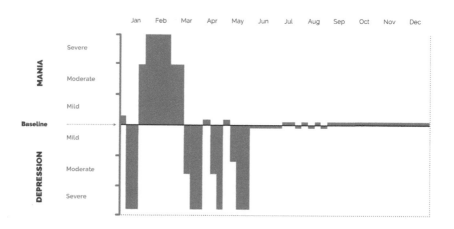

1-Year Life Chart – 2005

These charts were initially a tool for me (and those close to me) to understand, track, and potentially predict my illness and its related symptoms. However, once I began speaking in corporations and schools about my experiences in order to reduce the negative effects of mental illness, I realized the storytelling power of these images.

As a result, a portion of every keynote or seminar I deliver is dedicated to walking audiences through what these charts represent. They are also included in the programs available through The StigmaZero Online Training Academy. More than that, I explain how it felt to go through those dramatic and intense states and how much societal stigma added to the already daunting challenge.

I also share four strategies for managing my illness and maintaining the highest quality of life that my illness will allow. Here are the key ways I manage my illness:

- Energy Management
- Nutrition and Exercise
- Caregivers
- Medication

Energy Management

Long ago, I accepted the simple fact that because I have bipolar disorder, my energy levels are, at times, lower than average. This affects my stamina and capabilities, so I keep a regular seven- to eight-hour sleep schedule and never get less than seven hours on consecutive nights. Sometimes I decline social invitations, not because I don't want to go, but because I know I need rest to avoid crashing. And when I feel really worn out, I don't hesitate to take a day (or two) to completely recharge and reset. This has often saved me from sliding into a depressive episode.

Nutrition and Exercise

This one is easy. I eat reasonably well, get regular exercise, and drink plenty of water. I am by no means exceptional–my wife and many of our friends eat far more strictly and exercise far more than me. However, I have a fairly balanced diet and move as much as I can when my energy allows. My main passions of golf and curling help me do this. I know nutrition and exercise are important pieces of the puzzle.

Caregivers

Ninety-nine percent of the time, if someone is helping me manage my illness, it is my beautiful wife, Anna. Using a golf analogy, Anna is the best caddy I could ask for, helping me stay on track with these management strategies, pointing out when I slip, helping me notice energy level changes, and generally being patient. Others support me as well, and I don't feel guilty for accepting their help or Anna's.

Honestly, it feels like teamwork, not pity or charity. I know how lucky I am to be able to say all of that, and I never take it for granted. For anyone suffering from a mental illness, caregivers are important; you simply cannot do it alone.

Medication

This final method is no more or less important the others. I have been fortunate to respond well to medical treatments for bipolar disorder, and the two that work for me are lithium (which I have been taking since 2005) and escitalopram (also known as Cipralex, which I have been taking since 2012). These two treatments do a fantastic job of holding back the symptoms of bipolar: depression, hypomania, and mania. I never resent taking these medications or feel ashamed to do so.

Many people don't respond well to treatment like this and as a result have never found an effective strategy with medications. I know they'd love to be in my position. Each night as I take my medication, I feel gratitude.

RELATIONSHIPS TESTED, BROKEN, REPAIRED–AND FOUND

My Mom

I am fortunate I had the opportunity to express to Mom my under-standing of her struggle with mental illness, and ask her to forgive me for the years when I had stigmatized it. Although we had cathartic con-versations and, overall, my relationship with her was strong, challenges still came up from her ongoing illness and my need to manage my own.

The most dramatic example of this conflict involved my wedding to Anna in 2008. As we were preparing for our big day, I had a specific request for Mom—I needed her not to drink. *At all.*

At this stage of Mom's life, she wasn't well physically and was quite underweight. Although she didn't drink volumes and hadn't for years, the effect of one drink on her was like five drinks for most people. She would begin to slur, and she'd get tipsy. I didn't want to see or deal with these behaviors on my wedding day.

One day about five months before our big day, I told Mom, "I need you to not drink at my wedding; not one drink, not even a glass of champagne for the toast."

"What will others think?" she protested.

"I will have the servers keep your glass filled with non-alcoholic champagne, so no one but you or I will even know, Mom," I replied. "What matters is that I don't want to see you affected by alcohol on my wedding day."

To my surprise, she decided this wasn't a reasonable request and wouldn't promise me she'd avoid alcohol entirely. I let her know I was serious and that she wouldn't be welcome at the wedding unless she agreed. I gave her a few months to think about it.

One month before the big day, I checked in with her to see if she had changed her mind. I was saddened to hear she had not, knowing this meant I had to tell my own mother she wasn't welcome at our wedding. It was a hard conversation, but the simple reality was I had to take care of myself and my own health now that I was living with bipolar disorder. Planning a wedding is already stressful and demanding. I couldn't allow Mom's insistence on drinking alcohol to create more stress and anxiety for us.

I don't think she believed me initially, and she was quite upset when I made it clear I was serious and always had been. She had chosen her right to drink over attending her youngest son's wedding, which was incredibly sad and disappointing. This became an important lesson in knowing I can't control others, and also that I must set parameters in my own life. Those parameters will help me maintain my overall health and wellness while limiting the chance for relapses.

Naturally, this entire situation put a new strain on my relationship with Mom, although we were able to fully reconcile over the next few years. She ultimately realized she was wrong in her stance about my wedding, and she agreed it had been a fair request. Although I didn't need to hear that from her, I did appreciate it.

I'm also deeply thankful we were able to reconcile. In 2010, Mom was diagnosed with an aggressive form of nerve cancer. This illness proved too much for her frail body to handle. She declined quickly over six months, ultimately passing on May 6, 2011. Just two days before she died, I called the hospital to see how she was doing. To my surprise, I was connected directly to her, and we spoke for nearly ten minutes. Although she was being brave, we were both aware this was the likely the last time we would speak to each other.

It was a gift that many wish for but never get. I was able to remind her that, although it came late, I did finally come to understand her battle with mental illness and how her attempted suicide wasn't a selfish or hurtful act. Mom reiterated her regret for missing my and Anna's wedding and apologized again. We told each other how much we loved one another, and we said goodbye.

Because of the timing of her passing, my brothers and I planned her funeral service and burial on Mother's Day weekend. It was a terribly sad time, but we knew how she had suffered towards the end. We felt relieved she was finally at peace.

About a year before her passing, Mom had given me a letter containing instructions for her funeral. There were many small requests from the type of casket (pink) to the music we should play (Elvis, her favorite). We honored them all, of course. But there was one small request that we were surprised by, and it created a sweet moment and enduring memory for all of us.

Mom asked that her three boys release four pink balloons during the burial service, one for each of us and one for our sister, Tonia, who had died shortly after birth. There was something incredibly poignant and beautiful about standing over my mother's grave with my two older brothers, and simultaneously releasing the four pink balloons. We watched for a long moment as they floated up into the sky and eventually out of sight.

My Fiancée

In previous chapters, I referenced my fiancée several times. In the dedication at the start of the book and in this chapter, I mention my wife, Anna. It would be natural to assume they are the same person, but they are not. Here's what happened.

Although I was ultimately able to find an effective treatment for bipolar disorder and recover my health, my relationship with my fiancée was not as fortunate. The years of dramatic mood swings combined with the trauma of my manic episode had destroyed the foundation we had built together. She had offered me every ounce of support she could. But as I recovered my health, the toll on her became clear. I understood she couldn't live with the fear of it all happening again.

There was another major factor, as well. We had always planned to start a family once we were married, but my bipolar disorder forced me to reconsider that decision. I realized that to successfully manage my illness required a stable lifestyle with consistent sleep patterns—and having children would interfere with that. As anyone with children understands, the single biggest strain on regular sleep patterns is having kids. I realized it would almost certainly cause relapses, and I couldn't bear the thought of being a father who was too ill to fulfill the role. I had the luxury of choice in this major life decision, and I knew in my heart what I had to do.

So ultimately, bipolar disorder ended our seven-year relationship and two-year engagement. While we both felt sad, thankfully the split was amicable and went as smoothly as possible.

Suddenly Single

I must admit, however, that it was extremely lonely and scary to be suddenly single and living on my own. Considering I was recently diagnosed with bipolar disorder, hadn't been single in seven years, and didn't want children, how exactly should I approach dating?

At one particular moment, the reality of it all hit me. The movers had just finished unloading the truck and driven off. I was left standing in the middle of my new apartment, surrounded by boxes and completely alone. It felt like a wave crashing over me. Although the lithium was effective in treating my illness and I wasn't feeling any symptoms of bipolar disorder, in that moment, I felt the kind of crushing emotional depression anyone might feel after a loss of great magnitude. I could barely stand and definitely couldn't start the task of unpacking.

So I wiped away the tears, collected myself, and walked down the street to an internet café. Since nothing was set up in my apartment, going online was a way for me to connect with my family and friends and just distract myself. I stayed there for hours, not wanting to face my apartment. Eventually, I went back, headed straight to bed, and slept for twelve hours. After I woke up, I felt some relief, even a sense of hope, and began to unpack and set up my new apartment and my new life.

After a few months of settling in, I felt ready to at least try dating again. The only problem was I had no idea how. I wasn't the type to meet women in bars, and I saw no potential opportunities at work. I did, however, have several female friends and colleagues, so I started asking for their advice. How could a guy like me meet women?

One of my colleagues suggested online dating, but my initial reaction was negative. Thankfully, over the course of a few weeks, she persisted with the idea, even going so far as to suggest which dating website I should try: Lavalife. A friend of hers had used it with good experiences. She kept asking me, "Jason, what do you have to lose?"

An Online Dating Success Story

Eventually I saw this as my best option, so I set up a Lavalife account and created my profile. At the time, the idea of putting my image on a dating site felt weird to me, so I chose a photo that partially obscured my face. Given society's current level of comfort with putting out personal images, my modesty seems comical to me now! And here's the irony: By speaking publicly about my experiences with physical and mental illness, as well as founding StigmaZero and writing this book, I am more publicly known than I ever could have imagined at that time.

As I completed my profile, I made a decision that would prove to be key: I wrote my profile with as much attention to grammar and detail as I would write a cover letter and résumé. Combined with my obscured face in my profile picture, I went out of my way to ensure that anyone interested in me would be attracted because of what I said more than how I looked. And that's exactly what happened.

After nearly four years of struggle, challenge, disappointment, and loss, I caught the break of my life. I logged onto Lavalife one day in January 2006 and found a "smile" had been sent from someone called "SOCCERGIRL#2." ("Smiles" were the way to initially show interest in someone on Lavalife.) I looked at her profile and was immediately interested: smart, beautiful, clearly independent, and showing a strong personality. SOCCERGIRL#2 seemed to have it all.

We began chatting via Lavalife's text application and learned each other's real names. We also felt the chemistry between us, so we moved to MSN chat. (I feel like I am dating myself as young readers may not recognize what that is. MSN was the "Microsoft Network" chat service that allowed easy and free online chatting, very similar to WhatsApp today. It was shut down in 2013, after fourteen years on the market.) We had several days of long text conversations, revealing we had nearly everything in common—from music to movies to literature. After that, we set up our first date at Hurley's Irish Pub in downtown Montreal.

Our chemistry extended beyond the virtual. Anna and I hit it off immediately. In fact, our first date was an epic conversation that started at seven in the evening and wasn't over when Hurley's closed for the night. We continued our date by walking the downtown streets on an unusually warm February night. Anna finally dropped me off at home at five in the morning. As she drove away, I knew my life had just changed completely. It was the happiest I had felt in years.

All of this posed a problem for me, though. When your first date is that good, how long do you wait to tell that special woman you have a mental illness called bipolar disorder and you don't want children?

We were both thirty years old at the time, and I was aware how time was of the essence. If Anna wanted children or was uncomfortable being thrust into the role of a caregiver of someone with a mental illness, it wasn't fair to her to wait to tell her. But should I tell her on our second date? And if I *should* do it ... could I?

Second Date Chemistry

Soon after Anna arrived at my apartment for our second date, all of the attraction and chemistry from the first date picked up where it had left off. I felt like it was the hundredth time I was seeing her, not the second. I knew I couldn't wait to tell her.

I can't believe I found the courage to have that conversation and present not one but two possible deal-breakers. And I hated the thought of our adventure ending right then and there, but I had to tell her out of respect for her. That thought helped me to start the conversation.

"I don't want to get ahead of myself, but I have a few things I need to tell you, Anna ..."

Anna was amazing. After the initial wave of shock passed over her face, she listened and asked smart questions. Among them: What was bipolar disorder exactly? How would the symptoms return, if they ever did? What would you need in the way of support if they did? Why don't you want kids?

All of her questions came from an empathetic, neutral, and caring place. I will never forget that conversation; I knew how much was at stake.

Finally, after listening to me, asking her questions, and hearing my answers, Anna said two things that changed my life forever.

First: "The fact that you have bipolar disorder doesn't change how I feel about you or my interest in dating you. Just tell me what you need from me and know you can talk to me about anything."

Second: "As for not wanting children, several months ago, I came to the decision that I was open to either having my own children or not, depending on how life unfolded. If I met someone who desperately wanted his own kids and everything else was great, that would be fine with me. If I met someone who didn't want kids, I knew I'd also be fine with that. I like you and want to keep dating you, and the fact that you don't want kids doesn't change that."

In that moment, I felt like I'd won the lottery. I proposed on our first anniversary in February 2007 and we married on February 2, 2008.

CAREGIVER ANGELS

When it comes to illnesses like my heart defect or cancer, we intuitively understand the need for caregivers. By caregivers, I mean people in the lives of the person facing an illness who can provide regular emotional, physical, and practical support. Yes, doctors and nurses provide care; it's their job to do so. But we don't spend the majority of our time with them unless we are hospitalized. Thus, any effective support system includes caregivers who are either family or friends.

Mental illness also requires caregivers. The potential for stigma, denial, misconceptions, non-compliance with treatment, and other factors add a great deal of complexity.

I can say without question that caregivers have had a vital role in the successful management of my illness. First, my fiancée helped me ultimately overcome the stigma I felt towards mental illness. She also helped me learn about it and better manage it through mood and sleep tracking. Finally, she was instrumental in helping my family understand the severity of my manic episode before my behavior became destructive. I will forever be grateful for all the ways she was there for me.

After I met Anna, I was fortunate to live at my baseline for several years. The lithium was working, and so were my management strategies, with Anna providing critical support in that process. However, she was thrust into the role of caregiver in 2012 when I had a relapse of mild depression. That was followed by several episodes of moderate depression over the next few years. The following charts illustrate how my illness presented during those years:

> **Author's Note:** As in the changes from 2002–2005, "baseline" indicates my normal level of health, energy, and general function. Shading above or below the baseline indicates when I was experiencing the symptoms

related to the states labeled on the left. Mild and moderate mania are also known as "hypomania," while severe mania is known as "manic" or a "manic episode." Depression is generally categorized as mild, moderate, or severe. However, as mentioned, many people experience each of those states differently than I did.

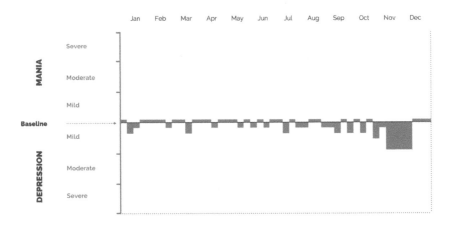

1-Year Life Chart – 2012

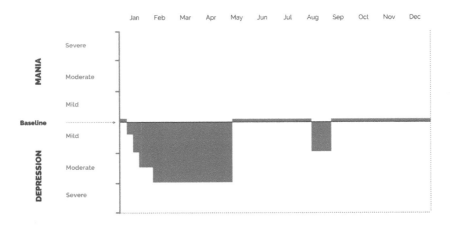

1-Year Life Chart – 2013

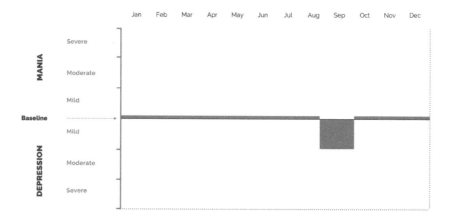

1-Year Life Chart – 2014

Adjustments

Ultimately, these relapses required adjusting and then adding to my treatment, a process that involved countless blood tests and visits with my doctors. I experienced new side effects, some of them quite terrible. Thankfully, they didn't last long, but overall, I faced a challenging period in my life. Without Anna's unwavering support—and total lack of stigma, judgment, and discrimination—my recovery would have been infinitely more difficult.

Throughout this process, my doctors and I discovered that lithium was no longer effective at treating both aspects of my bipolar disorder. While it had a perfect track record in preventing hypomania or mania, as my 2005 through 2014 charts show, I was experiencing more and more depressive episodes. Ultimately, my doctor prescribed a reduction in lithium (since less was required to prevent mania) and an additional treatment for depression: escitalopram.

I began taking escitalopram in April 2013. As the chart shows, it became dramatically effective in May that year. The side effects were unpleasant, including a week of feeling like my skin was crawling nonstop. But the side effects faded after six weeks or so, and I was grateful we had found a treatment that was working well.

The two depressive episodes noted in the charts in August 2013 and August 2014 occurred because my body was adapting to the new treatment and suddenly required a higher dosage. My doctor said this was quite common. After twice increasing my dosage by a small amount, the medication worked again. I have not had a significant depressive episode (defined as lasting for more than a few days) since September 2014. Also, since then I have remained at the same dosage of both lithium and escitalopram.

If you are a caregiver for someone with a mental illness, know that you are playing a crucial role, whether that person expresses it to you or not. Be proud of your generosity and empathy, and know your efforts have an immensely positive impact.

If you are someone who suffers from a mental illness, make sure you identify people in your life who are able to be caregivers for you. You cannot do this alone.

SPEAK UP AND FIGHT!

Once I fully owned my illness, I realized I had the opportunity to assist others by sharing my stories and insights. Experiencing both a major physical and mental illness provided the perspective; my background in theater and speech communication provided the ability.

So I started talking. I first approached a not-for-profit organization in Montreal called AMI Quebec, which supports caregivers of those with mental illness as well as delivers education services for local schools and companies. The AMI stands for Action on Mental Illness, and when I was learning about my own illness, I had taken a valuable "Mood and Thought Disorders" course at AMI Quebec. Because of that, I respected what the organization stood for. I wanted to help.

I volunteered to share my story as part of an education program delivered by AMI Quebec's educational coordinator. We co-presented in high schools, colleges, universities, and corporations. Since 2006 when I first volunteered, I've delivered close to forty presentations, key-notes, and training sessions on this topic to over 2,200 people for AMI Quebec alone.

The volunteer work I did from 2006 to 2012 was extremely forma-tive. Given my education in theater and speech communication, as well as the many opportunities I've had to present publicly, both socially and professionally, I knew I was a strong speaker. What I didn't know was if my story—and the manner in which I shared it—would have an impact on audiences.

As it turned out, that impact was far more than I could have imag-ined. Every single time after I've delivered a keynote speech or train-ing session, at least a few—and often several—audience members have shared with me how my story profoundly affected them. Often, they gained a new, deeper understanding of their own mental illness and/or stigma. Also, if they had never experienced a mental illness directly, my story helped them better see the people in their lives who were facing it. They realized they hadn't supported them in ways they would have if they'd had a physical illness. Stigma was holding back their own treatment or affecting how they supported a loved one.

Repeatedly, one of the most gratifying aspects of my work comes when people tell me I helped break down the stigma in their minds. They say they will now approach mental illness in a more proactive and healthy way.

THE GET-WELL CARD INCIDENT

As I have explained, bipolar disorder presents with symptoms of hypo-mania and mania "highs" as well as clinical depression "lows." For me, the depressions in particular were so severe I was incapable of working, so I was prescribed a medical leave of absence. Although my employer had an excellent HR staff as well as sick benefits to respond to the situation, my manager and colleagues were caught off guard.

In part because of my own stigma towards mental illness at the time, I was uncomfortable sharing why I needed to take a leave. As a result, my colleagues only knew I was sick and had to take a "medical leave of absence." Only my immediate manager knew details of my condition, which at the time was believed to be clinical depression.

The positive environment I worked in was filled with intelligent, well-educated, and empathetic individuals. I had been a part of the team for a few years and was well-known and liked—all the ingredients to have a positive support system during my leave and when I returned. But the powerful stigma that surrounded mental illness got the better of us. First, I felt the need to keep my illness secret, and second, my colleagues didn't know how to react. Their normal instincts didn't apply easily.

Which brings me to the "get-well card incident."

After several months of fighting my illness at home with zero contact from my employer, except for my manager and the HR case worker assigned to me, I received a get-well card. It was signed by all the members of my team as well as several other colleagues. It should have felt good to receive it, but it didn't. The fact that it came strangely late into my leave was one thing; the other was that they had only signed their first names. No comments, notes, or well-wishes were written—as if they didn't know what to say.

But that's only part one of the "get-well card incident." The second part came a few months later, after I had returned to work. Another colleague fell ill, this time with a serious virus that kept him in hospital for several weeks. We were all concerned, and naturally within a few days of him falling ill, someone organized a get-well card for everyone to sign. On a massive, oversized card, every square inch was filled with thoughtful notes and comments. They wished he'd get well and come back soon; they wrote that he was missed, that we were all pulling for him to recover.

I was glad to have the chance to sign the card and add my own note. I thought what everyone wrote, and the sheer size of the card, would lift his spirits. It felt great to contribute. Everything about it felt right, appropriate.

However, as I walked back to my office, I was overwhelmed by a surge of anger that seemed to come from nowhere. In fact, I was furious. It took me a while to realize I was reacting to the injustice of the two situations. *Why was his illness worthy of this fast, positive response, while mine was not? Why did everyone know the appropriate response to his physical illness but not to my mental illness?*

My anger wasn't directed at my colleagues for their response to my sick leave, nor was it at the timely, positive response given to our colleague in the hospital. I was angry that something as ridiculous and unnecessary as stigma could create such completely disparate responses to two similar situations. And I was disappointed in myself that I'd been a part of the problem, allowing self-stigma to guide my actions.

Self-stigma—applying the stigma commonly felt towards mental illness to oneself—is a dangerous trap for anyone experiencing a mental illness. When you feel ashamed, guilty, confused, and afraid of others' opinions about an illness you are facing, how are you supposed to respond in a healthy, pro-active way?

Situations like this "get-well card incident" are still common in workplaces, and in many cases, they lead directly to losses in productivity. That may not seem like an obvious outcome; however, when employees see overt examples of stigma towards mental illness in their workplace, it significantly changes their behavior if they experience the symptoms of such an illness.

For example, they are likely to delay seeking treatment, which results in presenteeism (when someone attempts to work through an illness rather than disclose it). In addition, if they do need to take a leave of absence as a result of mental illness, the return to work can be fraught with fear, discomfort, and a feeling they no longer belong.

In effect, this lack of support in cases of mental illness is costing billions each year, but it doesn't have to be this way. We can learn to respond to mental illness in the workplace in the same thoughtful way we already respond to absences caused by physical illnesses.

Stigma: Based on Fear and Lack of Understanding

My core message is that stigma around mental illness exists only because of fear and a lack of understanding. Stigma may well be innocent in its origin, but it doesn't belong.

When stigma exists in a person's mind, as it did in mine, it's difficult to change. I often use my creativity to get this point across, such as in this example.

A close friend struggled to understand that my bipolar disorder was an illness and not an "issue" rooted in my emotional self. In addition to the "issue" tag, he had used these familiar lines: "Can't you just try harder and snap out of it?" and, "Do you really need to take that medication?"

At one point, he began suffering from kidney stones. During one of our conversations, he complained that he had to drive for several hours to a clinic to have his kidney stones "zapped" so they could be passed. Seeing an opportunity, I asked him a few simple questions:

> Do you really *need* that treatment?
> Can't you just *try harder* and zap your kidney
> stones yourself?
> Are you sure you even need a doctor to help you with
> this "*issue?*"

After a long pause, he said, "Jason, I get it." And he never again spoke of my illness in any other terms than what it is—an illness.

During my keynote addresses, corporate workshops, as well as in the programs available in The StigmaZero Online Training Academy, I've consistently used metaphors to help break through the barrier in people's minds that allows stigma to exist and flourish. My experience tells me this is effective because it bridges the gap between people's impression of mental illness—often fed by negative and stigmatized media, stories, rumors, movies, television—and its reality. Once mental illness is presented in a way that makes sense in their experience of the world, real progress can be made.

Author's Note: Using metaphors can help people reach the same realization I had come to because of my heart defect and subsequent surgery. Now I often say, "Mental illness is an illness, like my heart defect was. It's not the fault of the person suffering. Like other well-known illnesses such as diabetes or cancer, there's no justification for any stigma, judgment, or discrimination."

CHAPTER 4
WHY STIGMAZERO?

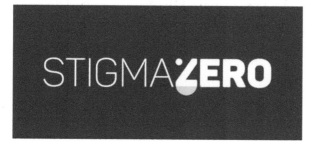

AN ORGANIC PROGRESSION

During the first seven years of doing presentations for AMI Quebec in Montreal, I continued to work full-time in my career as a fundraising and alumni relations professional. After I left McGill University, I worked for two private schools in Westmount, a suburb of downtown Montreal. I was giving about five volunteer presentations a year for AMI and was consistently improving my content and delivery. Given the positive reactions I was receiving, my message was clearly helping people better understand mental illness and stigma, which was a wonderful feeling.

Always supportive of my volunteer work, my wife Anna attended several of my presentations. Applying her strong business mind, she said, "You should really be doing this full time. I think you can make a living with this. And if you do it full time, you will reach so many more people."

Full time? For a living? This idea seemed radical to me.

However, over the next few years, we realized my passion and talent lay in this area. I wanted to do this full time, so it was only a matter of practicality. Once we decided we could take the risk, in January 2015, I officially became an entrepreneur.

As with any new venture, I needed to develop my services further to create my branding, so I spent the first two years doing exactly that. And with each new client, I developed my service offering, my mission, vision, value proposition and, ultimately, a new company name—StigmaZero. During this time, I realized I would need a partner to help me develop and grow the business. Rylan McKinley officially joined as Co-Founder and Head of Growth in 2017.

During these formative years, I completed extensive research, co-wrote a white paper establishing the ROI of investing in stigma reduction in the workplace, and developed a methodology to help employers address this challenge. This methodology was designed to address the unique and significant task of workplace culture change. I would train senior leadership and HR personnel first, then management, then employees.

After working in person to train clients on how they can change their culture and ultimately learn how to eradicate workplace stigma, it became clear that we needed a more efficient way to deliver our training. Over the course of 2018, Rylan and I worked towards building a new online training program. In order to make sure we did everything to the highest possible standard of quality, we surrounded ourselves with experts in the pedagogy of e-learning (Pure & Applied), design (Brandlucent), videography, editing, animation and design (5 Pound Media, HRVST), and web design (Brand Market Media).

The result is The StigmaZero Online Training Academy, which features our innovative and comprehensive *Create Your StigmaZero Workplace Program*, and can be found at www.StigmaZero.com.

ADDRESSING STIGMA IN THE WORKPLACE

Why People Hide Their Mental Illness

Each year for close to seventy years, the Canadian Mental Health Association (CMHA) has celebrated Mental Health Week. The theme one year was GET LOUD for mental health (#GETLOUD) and, like many other initiatives, the celebration week was intended to raise awareness and end discrimination surrounding mental illness.

Because of the stigma around mental illness, I have an acute understanding of the need for awareness campaigns. Through the *Create Your StigmaZero Workplace Program* offered in The StigmaZero Online Training Academy, I ask participants to complete a confidential survey. Their answers to two of the questions offer both a reason for hope, and a reminder that we still have work to do.

Question 1: Do you think people can control symptoms of a mental illness in the same way they would a bad mood or a stressful period in their lives?

In answering this question, the overwhelming majority of audience members respond "No," and add comments such as "They cannot control symptoms of a mental illness as they would a bad mood; it is an illness and requires treatment." This is evidence that a growing majority of people understand mental illness to be exactly that—an illness that requires treatment.

Question 2: If you were to experience symptoms of clinical depression or anxiety, would you be ashamed, feel guilty, and be likely to hide it from your colleagues, friends, and/or family? Or would you be comfortable to come forward?

Approximately sixty percent of responses to this second question indicate their first instinct would be to feel guilty, ashamed, fearful, and, ultimately, to hide the symptoms. They'd "soldier on" rather than come forward. Of those who responded in this way, the majority had indicated their understanding of mental illness in their answer to the first question.

This shines a light on the stigma that still affects people suffering from mental illness. Stigma is a powerful force, even for the people who already understand that mental illness is an illness.

We need to keep working together to address this challenge until everyone who suffers from a mental illness can proceed in the same way someone would after a cancer diagnosis. They could speak freely about their illness, seek help, and be unafraid of stigma, judgment, and discrimination.

Although we are on the right path, we aren't there yet.

CREATE YOUR
STIGMAZERO WORKPLACE
PART 5

Three Reasons to Address Workplace Stigma

Earlier in this book, I emphasized that "awareness isn't enough." Here are three reasons corporate leaders should address workplace stigma:

1. Mental illness is costly. In Canada, mental illness costs the economy an estimated $50 billion per year due to lost productivity, and it accounts for 40% of all disability claims. (*Source: Canadian Mental Health Association*)

   In the U.S., the impact is equally as staggering, as serious mental illness costs the U.S. economy $193.2 billion each year. (*Source: National Alliance on Mental Illness*)

2. Mental illness affects all levels of the organization.

   Nearly every corporate leader recognizes that mental illness is a major cause of lower revenues due to lost productivity. Corporations must face the challenge posed by mental illness on all levels: organizational, departmental, and individual.

   The *organization* faces loss of profits, risk of damaged reputation, and potential legal issues—to name just a few. The *department* must overcome the strains of workload management, the risk to employee morale, and the potential minefield of informal office communications. And in addition to a terrifying and potentially life-altering illness, the *individual* faces the daunting challenge of stigma.

3. We can't stop mental illness from affecting employees; we can, however, reduce and ultimately eradicate stigma.

   As with any other human resources challenge—from major physical illness to maternity leave—the most successful strategy focuses on what can be accomplished. For example, corporations can't (and shouldn't expect to) control employee absences caused by cancer or pregnancy. However, they typically implement policies to prepare for these eventualities and minimize any negative outcome.

What is the single strategy that will reap the most benefit? *Tackling stigma head-on.*

Awareness programs only scratch the surface. They fail to address the core problem, which is that stigma is deeply personal and it causes employees to behave differently towards themselves and others. Our *Create Your StigmaZero Workplace Program* found in The StigmaZero Online Training Academy is an effective first step towards reducing the stigma of mental illness. (You can find full details at www.StigmaZero.com.)

I encourage you to address the challenge of stigma with the goal of enjoying a healthier, more productive, and more profitable future.

THE IMPORTANCE OF EMPATHY

The more I consider what causes stigma regarding mental illness, and how we can eradicate it, the more I keep coming back to empathy.

Simply put, we do not stigmatize what we understand and therefore can feel empathy towards. This is why people who have illnesses such as a heart defect or cancer or diabetes suffer virtually zero stigma. Those around the person suffering see it as an illness that can't be controlled, and they are filled with empathy. They react to the person's illness swiftly with kind gestures such as phone calls and get-well cards.

That rarely happens with mental illness, and this can cause significant problems in the workplace. A commonly overlooked but crucial aspect to better managing mental illness is informal office communication. The "get-well card incident" shared earlier in this book is an excellent example of how important these informal communications can be.

How well do we understand empathy? The term is defined by the Oxford Dictionary as "the ability to understand and share the feelings of another."

When it comes to illnesses, we're able to instantly empathize with someone facing an illness like cancer, even when we've never experienced it. Why? Because our understanding of what cancer is and how it works is strong. We can imagine ourselves in the person's position, which leads to our ability to understand and share the feelings of another. In turn, it leads to a clear sense of how we would want to be treated in their position. This clarifies our own actions towards them.

However, with mental illness, this entire empathy process breaks down. If a person has never experienced the symptoms of a mental illness and has not been given any meaningful instruction on it, it's easy for them to have a lack of empathy. They don't understand what the person is going through, so they can't imagine how they would want to be treated in their place. This is the trap that leads to stigma.

The majority of employees, managers, and senior leadership personnel don't have a strong understanding of what mental illness is, the various ways it manifests, or even what stigma is and what causes it. So the first task for any employer who wishes to reduce, and ultimately eliminate, workplace stigma regarding mental illness is education and awareness.

When tackling stigma in the workplace—like tackling the sensitive, complex topics of racism and sexism—the right foundation must be laid to make a culture change. This culture change will affect how everyone in the organization understands, recognizes, and reacts to mental illness.

What is at the core? The language we use, both internally and externally, to address mental illness. (In Chapter 2, on pages 48-50, I reviewed the kind of hurtful, judgmental and stigmatized language that is so easily available to us because of media and pop culture—this is a good moment to go back and review the list of words provided.)

Five Common Traps to Avoid

Consider these five common traps to avoid when discussing mental illness:

1. Referring to mental illness as something the person suffering is *doing* rather than *experiencing*.

   This trap most commonly occurs when a person speaks of another's mental illness in vague terms such as "issue," "problem," or "difficulty." On their own, these terms seem innocuous. However, we don't say such things when referring to someone who has cancer or has had a heart attack. In those cases, we choose phrases such as "Nancy has been diagnosed with breast cancer," and "Frank is in hospital recovering from a heart attack."

   The language in these examples makes it clear those things *happened to* Nancy and Frank, and aren't their fault. If we were to say "Nancy is having cellular health issues," not only would that sound odd, but it would imply that Nancy has some choice or responsibility in the matter. This opens the door to judgment, stigma, and discrimination while closing the door to empathy.

2. Allowing feelings of awkwardness or discomfort take the lead when discussing mental illness.

We have all been there. It's difficult to know what to say to someone who just lost a loved one or who has been diagnosed with a serious illness. We often feel awkward in these situations, whether the illness is physical (like cancer) or mental (like clinical depression).

However, with known physical illnesses, there's an overwhelming instinct to feel empathetic and show it when we're in these uncomfortable situations. Invariably, people find a way to show their feelings, and it is clear they're not judging, discriminating, or being guided by stigma in any way. Unfortunately, this empathy loses out to awkwardness when speaking about mental illness. What's the result? Those suffering feel concerned about *your* lack of comfort when you should be showing concern and comfort for them.

3. Doing or saying nothing.

    This is a related trap to #2. When we're afraid of the awkwardness we feel, it's easier to say or do nothing when a friend or colleague suffers from a mental illness. This can feel safe, but it is a dangerous trap, because when everyone (or the majority) follows this path, the person suffering receives little support.

    An excellent example of this is the "get-well card incident," described earlier.

4. Questioning the motives or work ethic of the person suffering.

    Clinical depression is one of the most common mental illnesses, and yet is is often misunderstood. Anyone who has ever felt depressed (which is everyone) can fall into the trap of thinking he or she understands clinical depression. As a result, it's easy to say, "I've felt depressed and was able to work through it. That wasn't fun, but I did it. Why can't you?"

    When I initially experienced clinical depression, I had to face this obstacle frequently. It's a terrible feeling to have to explain and, worse, justify the illness that was shutting down my life. To be that ill and fight through it harder than I've ever fought anything—and fail—was beyond frustrating. To then have others question my work ethic or motives was devastating.

5. Ask if a person plans to stop treatment now that he or she feels better.

I have been speaking for years, sharing my experiences with bipolar disorder to help them overcome stigma and reduce the impact of mental illness. During that time, I've lost count of the number of times I have been asked if I plan to stop my treatment (or if I ever thought of doing so), given I live relatively symptom-free today.

I have never understood this question. Growing up, I had a friend with Type 1 Diabetes who had to take two insulin injections every single day. He seemed healthy, but even at ten years old, I never once considered asking Patrick if he planned to stop his injections. I understood he had an illness and needed this treatment to control his symptoms.

Of course, not every mental illness is as clear-cut in its treatment as diabetes. However, in many cases, the treatment addresses a chemical imbalance that cannot otherwise be controlled. To ask this question implies that it can, in fact, be controlled by the person—which goes back to trap #4.

Falling into these traps is, unfortunately, easy to do given the prevalence of stigma in our society. It can—and does—happen to the best-intentioned of us. I have seen volunteers who dedicate their time to raising awareness of mental illness and stigma fall into one or more of these traps. I have seen professionals who have a deep understanding of mental illness and zero stigma towards it, yet they also fall into one of these traps.

Add to that a consistently negative portrayal in movies, television, news, and pop culture. In many ways, years of direct and indirect forms of discrimination towards mental illness have set us up to fail our fellow human beings.

Right now, I challenge you to overcome and avoid these traps. The sooner we all do that, the sooner stigma will be part of the past.

Olympics and Mental Illness—
What We Can Learn from Athletes

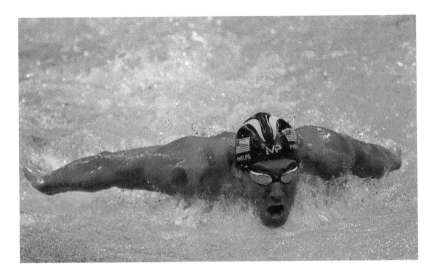

Photo credit: NBC Olympics

The human experience is often defined by successes and failures. Throughout our lives, each of us experiences memorable highs and painful lows. For many, the transition from one to the other can be made in a stable, healthy way without any lingering problems.

However, for those who are prone to a clinical mental illness such as depression, anxiety, or bipolar disorder, it is precisely these natural peaks and valleys that can trigger the symptoms of a real (and sometimes lasting) illness. The peak could be a major professional success, a financial windfall, or a personal milestone such as a marriage, anniversary, or addition to the family. The valley could be a death, a bankruptcy, a divorce, or the loss of a long-term job.

For an Olympic athlete, the very thing they train for—the Olympic Games themselves—can produce the loftiest of peaks and the deepest of valleys, all in a brutally short span of time. After years of training, these athletes must amp up the pace in the weeks leading up to the Games, and then produce a near super-human performance of focus and endurance under two weeks of extreme pressure.

But only a select few who aspire to bring home an Olympic medal have that dream fulfilled. Whether they win or not, the experience comes to a crashing halt the second the Games are finished. The transition to a standard pace of life can be treacherous—for both the winners and the losers. The challenge is adjusting from the extreme change in intensity of the Olympic experience to what feels like a mundane, "normal" life afterward. The term "post-Olympic depression" has been coined because it's so prevalent.

A well-known example of a world-class athlete facing post-Olympic depression is Michael Phelps, pictured in the photo. Despite being well on his way to be the most successful Olympian of all time, he suffered a serious depression after the 2008 Beijing Games. Many found his symptoms surprising; however, his story serves as a humbling reminder that mental illness can affect anyone.

For more detail on this topic, I encourage you to read John Florio and Ouisie Shapiro's insightful article "The Dark Side of Going for Olympic Gold" in the August 16, 2016, issue of *The Atlantic*. This article astutely highlights the challenge that stigma poses for these athletes, who are trained *not* to show weakness or ask for help.

In learning to live well with my own mental illness, bipolar disorder, a key strategy is to navigate my life's natural roller coaster of highs and lows. I don't try to eliminate them altogether—that is a fool's errand. However, I do recognize the threat they present to my wellness. During a particularly positive time, I have learned to anticipate and prepare for the eventual disappointment, or "crash," that so often follows. I maintain a steady sleep schedule, get regular exercise, and eat a healthy diet. The same strategy helps me recover when life presents a serious challenge, for example, the deaths of my mother and father-in-law.

I know that mental illness, whether it affects an Olympic athlete or the average person, requires attention, understanding, dedication, and focus. But it absolutely can be overcome if we break free from the stigma and fear surrounding it, and we ask for help.

The Most Overlooked Strategy to Boost Productivity and Morale

Many companies invest significant time and money in their employees' sense of morale and their productivity—as they should. Human beings are the most important resource any organization has. Often, their work has the most direct influence on bottom-line profits. Common examples of these investments include team building, skills training, improved cafeteria offerings, health and wellness programs, and more.

Although these initiatives are both important and valuable, even the most employee-centric company procrastinates in facing this growing challenge: workplace mental illness and the stigma that surrounds it.

Many employers recognize that mental illness is present in one out of four people, which means it's the most prevalent health challenge facing their workforce. Some employers address this challenge with awareness campaigns—a fantastic first step. But the underlying drawback is that employees do not disclose mental illnesses in the same way they do physical illnesses.

Clearly, it isn't the mental illnesses themselves but the stigma that handcuffs everyone involved. If an employee or manager were diagnosed with cancer, he or she would have no fear of judgment or reprisal in disclosing the illness and following a course of treatment. The same cannot be said if the illness were depression or anxiety.

Employees suffering with those illnesses often feel pressured to hide their symptoms, delay treatment, and soldier on.

Why is this true?

For the vast majority of workplace leaders, the topics of mental health and mental illness feel uncomfortable. They don't have the same tools, language, or experience to know how to respond. The resulting stigma creates enormous problems and has a tangible effect on productivity. What is the most significant consequence of stigma? Its silencing power. In turn, this causes presenteeism and greatly exaggerates the effect of the illness itself.

Challenges and Costs of Stigma in the Workplace

As business leaders increasingly recognize the challenges—and significant costs—due to mental illness in the workplace, they have begun investing in awareness programs, employee assistance plans (EAPs), and more. These initiatives indicate steps in the right direction and ingredients in any successful strategy; however, they often fail to address the core of the problem: stigma. But what does that really look like, and how can employers make dramatic improvements? I illustrate that in a series of graphics.

Figure 5 shows the series of challenges faced by an employee who has the misfortune of suffering from a mental illness:

Figure 5

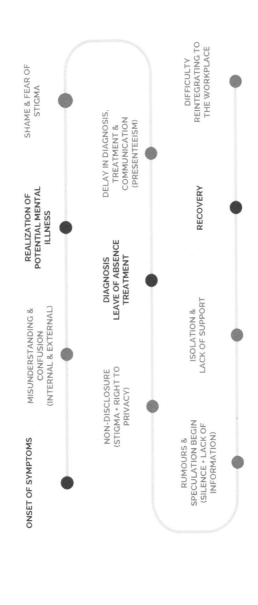

THE CHALLENGES FACED BY THE INDIVIDUAL EMPLOYEE

How stigma impacts the individual:

ONSET OF SYMPTOMS

MISUNDERSTANDING & CONFUSION (INTERNAL & EXTERNAL)

REALIZATION OF POTENTIAL MENTAL ILLNESS

SHAME & FEAR OF STIGMA

NON-DISCLOSURE (STIGMA + RIGHT TO PRIVACY)

DIAGNOSIS LEAVE OF ABSENCE TREATMENT

DELAY IN DIAGNOSIS, TREATMENT & COMMUNICATION (PRESENTEEISM)

RUMOURS & SPECULATION BEGIN (SILENCE + LACK OF INFORMATION)

ISOLATION & LACK OF SUPPORT

RECOVERY

DIFFICULTY REINTEGRATING TO THE WORKPLACE

As you can see, this is a daunting and largely unfair experience. Keep in mind, if the same employee is facing a diagnosis of cancer or other known illness, he or she is not forced to experience each of the steps shown in blue.

Figure 6 indicates the unnecessary steps in the current process. These steps exist only because of stigma.

Figure 6

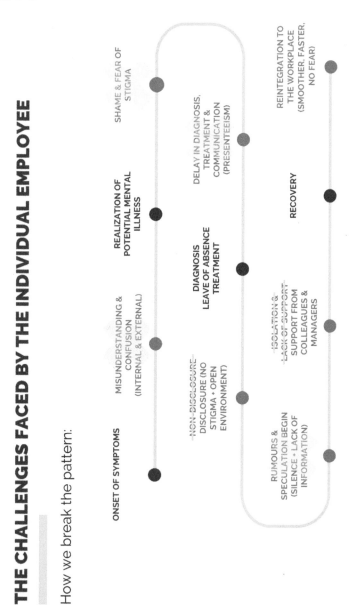

Once stigma is dramatically reduced and ultimately removed from the workplace, the same employee with the same mental illness diagnosis will have a dramatically improved experience, as shown in Figure 7.

Figure 7

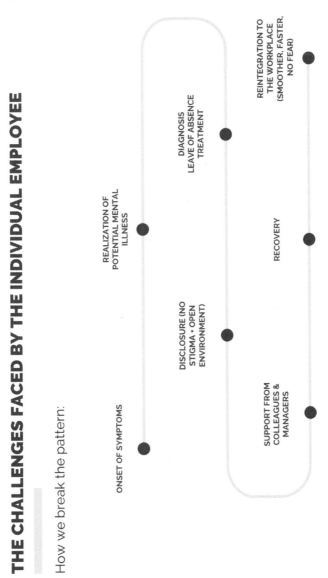

By investing in reducing workplace stigma, two main benefits will be realized:

1. Businesses will enjoy significant savings in the form of reduced losses caused by *absenteeism* and *presenteeism*— the two main drains on corporate profits caused by mental illness. (Presenteeism occurs when employees suffer from a mental illness but attempt to work through the illness due to fear of stigma and discrimination. These employees can work for extended periods at significantly reduced production levels before seeking treatment.)
2. Any employee facing challenges of a mental illness will enjoy the same rights, treatment, and respect as their colleagues with physical illnesses—without stigma.

All the support and awareness programs available cannot, on their own, reduce and ultimately eradicate stigma. To achieve this, employers must implement programs that directly address this unique challenge. You'll find the return on investment in doing so to be significant.

EPILOGUE

In the prologue of this book, I wrote: "Mental illness is unfair. It can tear apart relationships, ruin careers, and in the most tragic instances, it can end lives."

Unfortunately, this harsh truth continues to be a reality in today's society in general, and specifically in our workplaces. Yet we have the power to create real change by eradicating stigma, which in turn will improve things immensely for those who suffer from mental illness, as well as for their caregivers.

Stigma is entirely unnecessary. Born of fear and misunderstanding, it vastly complicates an already overwhelming challenge in our society. Ending stigma will have a profound effect on how someone responds to the onset of a mental illness. It will also affect how caregivers respond.

Ending stigma won't make suffering from mental illness go away. But without stigma, we can increase the chances of early detection, diagnosis, treatment, and recovery. Imagine how it could also reduce the instances of loneliness and despair that cause some people to die by suicide.

Yes, ending stigma can save lives.

Stigma Surrounding Breast Cancer?

It is absolutely possible for us to collectively end stigma, and I draw inspiration from the history of breast cancer. In the 1940s and '50s, a woman diagnosed with breast cancer had the misfortune of also facing social stigma, resulting in almost zero social support. To her, it would have been unimaginable that fifty years later, a wealth of unanimous support for breast cancer patients and research would exist. There would be rallies, walks, races, pink ribbons, denim days, girls for the cure—*and absolutely zero stigma*.

How did we end the stigma around breast cancer? The answer is awareness. And education. And recognizing that breast cancer is an illness that happens *to* people—*not* a failure on their part, *not* a character flaw, and *not* their fault.

We don't have stigma towards illnesses we understand. And there's no valid reason for us to have stigma towards mental illnesses, either. So let's level the playing field.

What Can We Do NOW?

I implore you to speak up about mental illness. That doesn't have to mean sharing your story publicly, as I have. If you have a stigma about your own illness or that of a loved one, reframe your thinking to see that it's a physical illness. The cause of the illness is neither your fault nor their fault.

I am passionate about the fact that we must all start treating mental illness with the same social constructs as we do with cancer or any other well-known physical illness. And if you are already free of stigma, I challenge you to be a leader socially and in your workplace, so you can help others do the same.

Let's ensure a future without stigma; a future in which stigma is regarded as totally unacceptable and out of place. We are heading in the right direction now, but collectively we have the power to accelerate the process and ensure we succeed.

I founded StigmaZero for the sole purpose of working towards a future without stigma. It may sound counterintuitive, but I hold out hope that, one day, the world won't need our services.

ACKNOWLEDGMENTS

Thank you to everyone who has extended a hand, free of judgment and stigma, during my long journey of living with mental illness. You treated me no differently than if I suffered a relapse of my heart defect, and your empathy was so appreciated. You helped to inspire me in founding StigmaZero and in writing this book.

I must thank several by name, starting with my wife, Anna. From our second date to this day, your unwavering support has been nothing short of astonishing. I am so lucky we found each other, and I am grateful for you every day. StigmaZero, this book, and a healthy version of me would not exist without your belief, support and encouragement—and your patience as I built my new business from the ground up.

Thank you to my family: Dad and Shirley, Sean and Lynne, Trevor, and Mom. You supported me through depression, hypomania, and a manic episode. You were forced to make the painful decision to have me hospitalized against my will. I know how hard that was, but despite how terrible it must have felt, you did me a great service that day. And since I found effective treatment and began living well despite bipolar disorder, your support has continued.

Thank you to my second family: Hanna and Zbigniew, and Peter and Alex. You never hesitated when you learned your daughter, sister and sister-in-law was dating someone with bipolar disorder. Even though you didn't have extensive knowledge of mental illness, you judged me for my actions and not my illness, and always made me feel completely welcome.

Before developing this business, I worked as a volunteer for many years for a Montreal-based support organization called AMI Quebec. It specializes in outreach education on mental illness and support for caregivers of those impacted. Thank you to all the coordinators at AMI with whom I worked over the years, and in particular Lori and Jillian. It was a pleasure working with you both as I was laying the foundation for StigmaZero. I would also like to acknowledge Mike, the first person I had seen share his story to help those coming to terms with their mental illnesses. You inspired me to follow in your footsteps, Mike–thank you.

When I first took the leap as an entrepreneur, I invited the smartest people I knew to dinner so I could share my new business ideas and collect their opinions and advice. Thank you to Anna, Jenn, Anita, Liz, and Melissa for all you offered that night, and for your unwavering support ever since. My decision to write this book was actually cemented that night when Anita raised the idea and the rest of you emphatically agreed it would be worthwhile. That meant a lot to me, and I will always be grateful.

Thank you to my Canadian Association of Professional Speakers (CAPS) colleagues for constantly inspiring me with your work. You have helped me shape my business and my message, as well as hone my platform skills. There are too many to thank everyone by name, but I would like to give special thanks to Toni and Ger, Nabil and Sylvie, Suzannah, Glynis, Bear, Marc-Antoine, Frema, Carol, Codi, Sandeep, Mark and Sarah for believing in me and the importance of my message.

Thank you to Kevin for generously offering me your mentorship; the guidance you have given me has been invaluable, as has been your uncanny ability to create meaningful connections with others in your network. You believed in me and StigmaZero from the very beginning, and I am forever grateful.

Thank you to Vic for your unwavering support and cheerleading over the past several years. You introduced me to Karen at Brandlucent, which proved to be an important connection, and always believed in the value of the work I am trying to do.

Thank you to Niki and Roxanne from Pure & Applied for your incredibly valuable input and guidance on this book, as well as your expert consultation, research and learning design work as we built The StigmaZero Online Training Academy and the *Create Your StigmaZero Workplace* Program. It has been a pleasure working with you, and I hope we can collaborate again on future projects.

Thank you to Karen from Brandlucent for being such an important part of my journey from the very beginning; your keen branding, marketing and design skills have resulted in a brand identity for StigmaZero that is evident throughout this book, our website and the StigmaZero Online Training Academy—and of which I am so proud.

Thank you to my book team: Barbara McNichol for her thoughtful and highly skilled editing services; and everyone at FriesenPress for their outstanding guidance and service every step of the way—in particular Bret, Miko, Jacob, Sarah, Diane and Oriana.

Thank you to Fany Ducharme (www.fanyducharme.ca) for your expert photography work on the cover photo as well as my "About the Author" headshot. You are a master of composition and light, and a delight to work with.

Thank you to Heather for reading an early draft of this book. Your feedback was so meaningful to me; in fact, the handwritten note you gave me is a treasured keepsake of this entire process.

Finally, thank you to Rylan, my friend and StigmaZero co-founder. You had a vision for StigmaZero that far exceeded my own, and I will be forever grateful for your belief in me and what I was doing. You also helped me get started on writing this book, and your feedback on an early draft was incredibly impactful on the final result. It is always a pleasure to work with you, and I am proud of the team we have become.

RECOMMENDED RESOURCES

Canadian Mental Health Association (CMHA)	www.cmha.ca
Centre for Addiction and Mental Health (CAMH)	www.camh.ca
Mental Health Commission of Canada (MHCC)	www.mentalhealthcommission.ca
Movement for Global Mental Health (MGMH)	www.globalmentalhealth.org
National Alliance on Mental Illness (NAMI)	www.nami.org
National Institute of Mental Health (NIMH)	www.nimh.nih.gov
World Federation for Mental Health (WFMH)	wfmh.global
World Health Organization (WHO)	www.who.int

GLOSSARY

Anxiety Disorder *National Institute of Mental Health (NIMH)*	Occasional anxiety is an expected part of life. You might feel anxious when faced with a problem at work, before taking a test, or before making an important decision. But anxiety disorders involve more than temporary worry or fear. For a person with an anxiety disorder, the anxiety does not go away and can get worse over time. The symptoms can interfere with daily activities such as job performance, school work, and relationships. There are several types of anxiety disorders, including generalized anxiety disorder, panic disorder, and various phobia-related disorders.
Bipolar Disorder *Centre for Addiction and Mental Health (CAMH)*	Bipolar disorder is a medical condition characterized by extreme mood swings that affect how people think, behave, and function. It causes a person to cycle through periods of depression and elevated mood swings. Bipolar disorder typically consists of three states: 1) a high state, called mania; 2) a low state, called depression; and 3) a well state, during which many people feel normal and function well. All people experience emotional ups and downs, but the mood swings for people with bipolar disorder are often more extreme.
Borderline Personality Disorder	Borderline personality disorder is a mental illness marked by an ongoing pattern of varying moods, self-image, and behavior. These symptoms often result in impulsive actions and problems in relationships. People with borderline personality

National Institute of Mental Health (NIMH)	disorder may experience intense episodes of anger, depression, and anxiety that can last from a few hours to days.
Depression, or Clinical Depression *World Health Organization (WHO)*	Depression is a common mental disorder characterized by persistent sadness and a loss of interest in activities that you normally enjoy, accompanied by an inability to carry out daily activities, for at least two weeks. In addition, people with depression normally have several of the following: a loss of energy; a change in appetite; sleeping more or less; anxiety; reduced concentration; indecisiveness; restlessness; feelings of worthlessness, guilt, or hopelessness; and thoughts of self-harm or suicide. Depression is treatable with talking therapies or antidepressant medication or a combination of these.
Hypomania & Mania *National Alliance on Mental Illness (NAMI)*	To be diagnosed with bipolar disorder, a person must have experienced at least one episode of mania or hypomania. Hypomania is a milder form of mania that doesn't include psychotic episodes. People with hypomania can often function well in social situations or at work. Some people with bipolar disorder will have episodes of mania or hypomania many times throughout their life; others may experience them only rarely. Although someone with bipolar may find an elevated mood of mania appealing—especially if it occurs after depression—the "high" does not stop at a comfortable or controllable level. Moods can rapidly become more irritable, behavior more unpredictable and judgment more impaired. During periods of mania, people frequently behave impulsively, make reckless decisions and take unusual risks. Most of the time, people in manic states are unaware of the negative consequences of their

actions. With bipolar disorder, suicide is an ever-present danger, because some people become suicidal even in manic states. Learning from prior episodes what kinds of behavior signals "red flags" of manic behavior can help manage the symptoms of the illness.

Mental Health *World Health Organization (WHO)*	Mental health is defined as a state of well-being in which every individual realizes his or her own potential, can cope with the normal stresses of life, can work productively and fruitfully, and is able to contribute to her or his community.
Mental Illness *World Health Organization (WHO)*	Mental illnesses, also known as mental disorders, comprise a broad range of health problems with different symptoms. However, they are generally characterized by some combination of abnormal thoughts, emotions, behavior, and relationships with others. Examples are schizophrenia, depression, intellectual disabilities, and disorders due to drug abuse. Most of these disorders can be successfully treated.
Obsessive-Compulsive Disorder (OCD) *National Institute of Mental Health (NIMH)*	Obsessive-Compulsive Disorder (OCD) is a common, chronic, and long-lasting disorder in which a person has uncontrollable, reoccurring thoughts (obsessions) and behaviors (compulsions) that he or she feels the urge to repeat over and over.
Schizophrenia *National Institute of Mental Health (NIMH)*	Schizophrenia is a chronic and severe mental disorder that affects how a person thinks, feels, and behaves. People with schizophrenia may seem like they have lost touch with reality. Although schizophrenia is not as common as other mental disorders, the symptoms can be very disabling.

Post-Partum Depression *National Institute of Mental Health (NIMH)*	Postpartum depression is a mood disorder that can affect women after childbirth. Mothers with postpartum depression experience feelings of extreme sadness, anxiety, and exhaustion that may make it difficult for them to complete daily care activities for themselves or for others. Postpartum depression does not have a single cause, but likely results from a combination of physical and emotional factors. Postpartum depression does not occur because of something a mother does or does not do. After childbirth, the levels of hormones (estrogen and progesterone) in a woman's body quickly drop. This leads to chemical changes in her brain that may trigger mood swings. In addition, many mothers are unable to get the rest they need to fully recover from giving birth. Constant sleep deprivation can lead to physical discomfort and exhaustion, which can contribute to the symptoms of postpartum depression. Some of the more common symptoms a woman may experience include: feeling sad, hopeless, empty, or overwhelmed; crying more often than usual or for no apparent reason; having trouble concentrating, remembering details, and making decisions; suffering from physical aches and pains, including frequent headaches, stomach problems, and muscle pain; persistently doubting her ability to care for her baby; and thinking about harming herself or her baby.
Self-Stigma *Oxford Dictionary*	Self-stigma exists at the individual level and involves the perceptions and experiences of those who possess stigmatized attributes. Individuals with stereotyped characteristics such as a mental illness are socialized into believing that they are devalued members of society, which leads to adopting negative feelings about self, engaging in maladaptive behavior, and identity transformation.

Individuals who feel devalued tend to modify their social expectations such that they settle into their low social position; they may not seek to advance their social status (either through education or work) or they may be reluctant to challenge the barriers standing in their way to a better life. Research indicates that mental illness-related self-stigma is associated with hopelessness, poorer self-esteem, disempowerment, reduced self-efficacy, and decreased quality of life.

Stigma *Oxford Dictionary*	A mark of disgrace associated with a particular circumstance, quality, or person. Synonyms: shame, disgrace, dishonor, humiliation, and bad reputation.
StigmaZero *Jason Finucan, Founder, StigmaZero*	The company founded by Jason Finucan and co-founded by Rylan McKinley, which has a vision of a future without stigma and a mission to help employers eliminate stigma in the workplace. In addition to keynote lectures by Jason Finucan, StigmaZero offers The StigmaZero Online Training Academy which includes the comprehensive *Create Your StigmaZero Workplace Program* to help employers better respond to mental illness in the workplace. Visit www.StigmaZero.com for more details.

STIGMA**ZERO**

empowering change.

ABOUT THE AUTHOR

Mental health advocate, stigma fighter, professional speaker and founder of the company StigmaZero, Jason is also the instructor of the StigmaZero Online Training Academy, which features the comprehensive program *Create Your StigmaZero Workplace* and can be found at www.stigmazero.com.

As someone who has experienced both a major physical illness (heart defect leading to open-heart surgery in 1988) and a major mental illness (bipolar disorder leading to hospitalization in 2005), Jason shares his personal experiences, both in this book and through his keynotes, with impactful storytelling techniques.

In order to make this difficult topic accessible and consumable, Jason blends his stories with rigorous research to mobilize knowledge and perspective. His goal is for everyone to understand this important topic so they are empowered to make a real change and ultimately join his vision for a future without stigma.

This is a mental health movement – and Jason wants you to be a part of it.

StigmaZero

Founded by Jason Finucan and Co-Founded by Rylan McKinley, who also serves as Head of Growth, StigmaZero offers a unique set of solutions to employers looking to improve their response to workplace mental illness, including:

- The StigmaZero Online Training Academy, which features the comprehensive program *Create Your StigmaZero Workplace*
- Keynotes by StigmaZero, through which StigmaZero Founder, Jason Finucan, is available to deliver high-impact keynote addresses, including his signature keynote Jason: 1, Stigma: 0
- On-site diagnostic, evaluation and consultation services, as needed

StigmaZero's mission is to help employers eliminate stigma in the workplace. As an organization, we share Jason's vision of a future without stigma while striking a balance between his advocacy, personal experience and storytelling and an academic approach. This includes rigorous research with the most current data and best practices regarding workplace mental illness and stigma.

Visit www.stigmazero.com for more information.